Access to Hea...

What does 'access to health care' mean? To what extent can we have truly universal, comprehensive and timely health services which are equally available to all? *Access to Health Care* considers the meaning of 'access' in health care and examines the theoretical issues that underpin these questions in health research and health policy.

Contributors draw on a range of disciplinary perspectives to investigate key aspects of access, including:

- geographical accessibility of services
- socio-economic equity of access
- patients' help-seeking behaviour
- organisational problems and access
- financial barriers and incentives to access
- methods for evaluating access.

Access is considered in both a UK and an international context. The book includes chapters on contrasting health policies in the United States and the European Union.

Access to Health Care provides health care researchers, as well as health professionals, managers and policy analysts, with a clear and wide-ranging overview of topical and controversial questions in health policy and health services organisation and delivery.

Martin Gulliford is Senior Lecturer in Public Health and **Myfanwy Morgan** is Reader in Sociology of Health in the Department of Public Health Sciences, King's College London.

Access to Health Care

Edited by Martin Gulliford
and Myfanwy Morgan

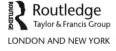
Routledge
Taylor & Francis Group

LONDON AND NEW YORK

First published 2003
by Routledge
11 New Fetter Lane, London EC4P 4EE

Simultaneously published in the USA and Canada
by Routledge
29 West 35th Street, New York, NY 10001

Routledge is an imprint of the Taylor & Francis Group

Typeset in Times by
HWA Text and Data Management, Tunbridge Wells
Printed and bound in Great Britain by
MPG Books Ltd, Bodmin

British Library Cataloguing in Publication Data
A catalogue record for this book is available from the British Library

Library of Congress Cataloging in Publication Data
A catalog record for this book has been requested

ISBN 0–415–27545–8 (hbk)
ISBN 0–415–27546–6 (pbk)

Contents

Contributors

Roger Beech is a Senior Lecturer in Health Operational Research, having joined the Centre for Health Planning and Management, Keele University, in 1998. Before that he held a similar position for 14 years in the Department of Public Health Medicine, GKT School of Medicine. His research and teaching concerns the planning and evaluation of health services, and the development of methodologies to help health professionals to undertake these tasks.

Sarah C. Blake is an associate faculty member at the Rollins School of Public Health at Emory University. Previously Sarah was a Research Scientist at the George Washington University's Center for Health Services Research and Policy in Washington, DC. Her work focuses on the delivery and financing of health care for underserved populations and women's health. She holds a Bachelor's degree in International Relations and a Master's degree in Public Policy.

José Figueroa-Muñoz is a Public Health Specialist Registrar and Honorary Lecturer in Public Health at Guy's, King's and St Thomas' School of Medicine, London. Having obtained a BSc in microbiology, he qualified in medicine in 1986 in Colombia and he then trained for a PhD in Medical Mycology at the St John's Institute of Dermatology, Guy's Hospital, London. Dr Figueroa's interest in epidemiology developed through research into the dermatological needs of tropical rural communities in South West Ethiopia. Dr Figueroa has a wide range of research interests relating to epidemiology of parasitic and infectious diseases, health inequalities, social determinants of health, community development and participation. He is a fellow of the Royal Society of Tropical Medicine and Hygiene, the British Epidermo-Epidemiology Society, and the British Society of Medical Mycology.

Barry Gibson is Lecturer in Sociology and Informatics as Applied to Dentistry at Guy's, King's and St Thomas' Dental Institute. Barry Gibson graduated from the University of Ulster with a first class honours degree in Sociology. He has an MSc in Paediatric and Preventive Dentistry and a PhD in Sociology as Applied to Dentistry from the Queen's University of Belfast.

Martin Gulliford is Senior Lecturer in Public Health Medicine in the Department of Public Health Sciences at King's College, London. He studied medicine at the University of Cambridge and University College Hospital, London. After working in the NHS, he trained in public health at Guy's and St Thomas' Medical School, London. His interests are in epidemiology as applied to health services research.

Robin Haynes is a Reader in the School of Environmental Sciences, University of East Anglia, where he was formerly a Lecturer and Senior Lecturer. He studied geography at the University of Bristol and Pennsylvania State University.

Kelly G. Howell is a Research Project Manager at the Emory Center on Health Outcomes and Quality. Previously she has worked as a microbiologist and as an infectious disease surveillance officer. She has an MPH in Epidemiology from the Rollins School of Public Health and a BS in biology from Virginia Polytechnic Institute and State University.

Meryl Hudson studied economics and geography at Queen Mary College, London, (1977). She then trained as a nurse at the Royal London Hospital (1979). Subsequently she has been involved with many different health service research projects for health authorities and the Universities of Surrey, Nottingham and King's College, London. She also continues with some clinical work.

David Hughes is an economic adviser at the Department of Health. Previously David was Senior Lecturer in Health Economics at the London School of Economics and King's College, London. He has also worked in Hong Kong as Economic Adviser and Assistant Professor at Hong Kong University School of Medicine. He has a first degree in Economics, an MSc in Health Economics from the University of York where he graduated with distinction, and a PhD in Economics from City University, London.

Myfanwy Morgan is Reader in Sociology of Health in the Department of Public Health Sciences at King's College, London. She studied at the University of London and University of Massachusetts, USA, and has previously held posts at the Department of Health and the University of Kent. Her research mainly focuses on the meanings and management of illness among patients from different socio-economic and ethnic groups, the evaluation of innovations in service delivery, and methodological issues relating to qualitative research.

Elias Mossialos is Brian Abel-Smith Reader in European Health Policy in the Department of Social Policy at the London School of Economics and Political Science, and Co-Director of LSE Health and Social Care. His research interests focus on comparative health policy, addressing questions related to funding health care, EC law and policy-making, cost-containment and private health insurance.

Sarah Thomson is Research Associate in Health Policy at LSE Health and Social Care (a research centre at the London School of Economics and Political Science) and Research Officer with the European Observatory on Health Care Systems.

Kenneth E. Thorpe is Robert W. Woodruff Professor and Chair of the Department of Health Policy and Management, in the Rollins School of Public Health of Emory University, Atlanta, Georgia. He was previously Professor of Health Policy and Administration at the University of North Carolina at Chapel Hill, and an Associate Professor and Director of the Program on Health Care Financing and Insurance at the Harvard University School of Public Health. Professor Thorpe was Deputy Assistant Secretary for Health Policy in the US Department of Health and Human Services from 1993 to 1995. In this capacity, he coordinated all financial estimates and programme impacts of President Clinton's health care reform proposals for the White House. As an academic, he has testified before several committees in the US Senate and House on health care reform and insurance issues.

Acknowledgements

The authors acknowledge the role of the NHS Research and Development Service Delivery and Organisation Programme in identifying 'access to health care' as a subject for investigation, and for supporting a preliminary review which led on to the writing of this book. A few sections of material in this book were included in the report, *Access to Health Care: A Scoping Exercise*. London: NHS R&D SDO Programme, 2001, which can be accessed from http://www.sdo.lshtm.ac.uk/access.htm. However, the views expressed in this book are those of the authors and not the funders. We also thank the editors and publishers of the *Journal of Health Services Research and Policy* for permission to reproduce an adapted version of 'What does "access to health care" mean?' from *Journal of Health Services Research and Policy* 2002, 7: 186–8. Finally, we thank Nike Williams for assistance in preparing the manuscript.

Chapter 1

Introduction
Meaning of 'access' in health care[1]

*Martin Gulliford, José Figueroa-Muñoz
and Myfanwy Morgan*

Introduction

Access to health care contributes to the improvement of health and the relief of sickness. In low-income countries problems of access concern the availability of basic health services such as the ability to visit a doctor or to receive health care during pregnancy and delivery. In affluent countries where basic services are generally accessible, questions of access concern the degree of comprehensiveness that can be offered by health care systems, the extent to which equity is achieved, and the timeliness and outcomes of care.

Access to health care has been justified in economic terms through its benefits in improving the health of entire communities, leading to conditions that favour economic growth (World Bank 1993). This utilitarian, efficiency-driven approach may not be sufficient to ensure that the needs of vulnerable or excluded individuals, such as the very old, people with mental health problems, or prisoners, are met. Access to health care has therefore come to be regarded as a basic human right and social goal in the sense that all individuals are considered to be entitled to health care, even though consideration of the economic benefit of the wider community does not necessarily require that they should receive it (Dworkin 1977). This is recognised by the United Nations in its Covenant on Economic, Social and Cultural Rights which recognises 'the right of everyone to the enjoyment of the highest attainable standard of physical and mental health' and requires governments to create 'conditions which would assure all medical service and medical attention in the event of sickness' (Office of the High Commissioner for Human Rights 1996: Article 12). In the Universal Declaration of Human Rights the rights to health and health care are set in a wider context which acknowledges the social determinants of health. Thus 'everyone has the right to a standard of living adequate for the health and well-being of himself and his family, including food, clothing, housing and medical care and necessary social services, and the right to security in the event of unemployment, sickness, disability, widowhood, old age or other lack of livelihood in circumstances beyond his control' (United Nations 1948: Article 25). Even in the United States, where access to health care is least secure among affluent countries, an amendment to the constitution has been proposed stating that 'all citizens and other residents of the United States shall have equal access to basic and essential health care' (Davidoff and Reinecke 1999: 692).

The United Nations' approach identifies health as a basic human right. This right focuses attention on a number of rights related to the conditions necessary for promoting and protecting health. These include protecting people from violence and inhuman and degrading treatment, promoting conditions of life and lifestyles that reduce risks of disease, injury and accident, as well as providing access to preventive and curative health services. In the European Convention on Human Rights, which was incorporated into United Kingdom law in the Human Rights Act of 1998, there is no explicit 'right to health', but the 'right to life' has been interpreted as requiring that all necessary health care should be provided (Thomson *et al.* 2001). Daniels (1985) attributes the right to health care to the importance of health in achieving normal human functioning, so access to health care is therefore a prerequisite for equality of opportunity in society. From this perspective a right to health care derives from the right to equality of opportunity.

Opposing arguments have been based on a particular view of the right to individual freedom. Thus a narrow libertarian view, which opposes a universal right to health care, has been expressed in these terms.

> Government can disguise the process by taxing the citizenry to reimburse the physician, pharmacy, and hospital. But the assault on the concepts of liberty and the pursuit of happiness is just as egregious. When their money is taken from them to pay for other people's health care, people's range of choices – that is, their freedom – is diminished.
>
> (Hornberger 2000)

This ideological debate concerning the appropriate role of the government in welfare and the nature of welfare policies is reflected in the approaches to the provision of health care in different countries (Deakin 1994). There are variations in the extent to which health care is seen as a public good, involving redistributive principles through tax-based or social insurance systems, or a largely private good which remains the responsibility of individuals. It follows that the contribution of private expenditures, and the roles of public and private sector provision of services, will also vary.

A basic assumption underpinning the public funding and provision of individual health services is that health care, and specifically medical care, is an important determinant of health. However, since the 1970s it has been increasingly acknowledged that medical care does not guarantee health. Indeed, medical care may in some instances form a cause of ill health through clinical iatrogenesis, including hospital-acquired infections or adverse and unanticipated side effects of drugs. For many conditions medical care is not the major determinant of health. More important factors include wider public health measures to reduce water and airborne diseases, health and safety at work, the reduction of environmental pollution, good nutrition and health-promoting behaviours in terms of exercise, smoking, drinking and sexual behaviour. The social and environmental determinants of health are differentially distributed in society, with some groups experiencing poorer health and having greater health needs. These inequalities in health must thus be addressed by wider public policy measures aimed at reducing poverty, and providing better education, employment conditions, housing, transport or nutrition (Acheson 1998). Despite this, timely receipt of health care has been shown to make a difference to health outcomes, particularly when assessed in terms of morbidity and broader measures of quality of life (Bunker *et al.* 1994).

Health care has a more specific value that is not fully measured in terms of improving health. The first lines of the 1983 report, *Securing Access to Health Care* by the President's Commission for the Study of Ethical Problems in Medicine and Biomedical Behavioural Research (1983) stated:

> The prevention of death and disability, the relief of pain and suffering, the restoration of functioning: these are the aims of health care. Beyond its tangible benefits, health care touches on countless important and in some ways mysterious aspects of personal life and invest it with significant value as a thing in itself.
>
> (p. 1)

As well as improved health and well-being, health care provides information about diagnosis and prognosis, and health care is intimately concerned with how people's lives will begin and end, and what opportunities they will have in between.

Health systems differ in the priority they give to universal access to health care. In the UK, a central principle of the National Health Service (NHS) in 1948 was the creation of a centrally funded system with universal eligibility to health care based on medical need, thus emphasising equity in terms of equal access for equal need. The NHS also aspired to comprehensive provision of care 'from cradle to grave'. By contrast in the US, health care is treated more like other goods and mainly allocated on the basis of ability to pay, but supported by a system of safety net public provision of basic health services to cater for those who are not able to meet this criterion of service use. These differences in approach to health care are shaped by wider economic and political forces, historical circumstances and cultural values. The NHS is firmly embedded within the philosophy of a welfare state which embraces notions of solidarity, with all citizens regarded as having rights to health, education and relief from poverty. In contrast, more market-oriented systems emphasise individual responsibility for health care. Increasingly health systems reflect a mix of public and market-oriented philosophies and practices.

Important questions which influence access to health care concern how health care should be funded and, if health care is not to be allocated according to price, how it should be distributed. The mechanisms put in place to ensure that health care is appropriately distributed will then determine who gains access to health care. The UK NHS developed from a consensus that health care should be financed according to ability to pay, but distributed according to need. Equity, in terms of equal access for equal need, became a key objective of the health system. In the US, the President's Commission (1983) argued 'that all citizens [should] be able to secure an adequate level of care without excessive burdens' (p. 4). Once these aims have been identified, there are difficulties involved in defining them more closely, and also in organising services that will deliver them. These practical problems form the main subject of this book.

In the UK, continuing public concerns about difficulties in gaining access to health care have led to two major programmes of health service reform in the last 15 years. Problems include delays in obtaining urgent appointments to see a primary care doctor, long waits for elective surgery, long waiting times in hospital accident and emergency departments, and difficulties accessing intensive care beds. Services sometimes seem not to meet adequately the requirement of groups with special needs. Some groups, such as old people, especially people with mental impairments and their carers, or people in institutions, may find that services are relatively inaccessible. For other groups, such as patients with sickle cell disease, services may not be sensitive to their requirements (Maxwell *et al.* 1999). There are also ongoing concerns about seemingly arbitrary geographical variations in access to health care, and wide social inequalities in health. In responding to these concerns, the UK government proposed that in future 'patients will get fair access to consistently high quality, prompt and accessible services right across the country' (NHS Executive 2001).

These concerns are widely shared. A recent survey of citizens' views in Australia, Canada, New Zealand, the United Kingdom and the United States found that more than half of respondents were dissatisfied with their health services and thought that fundamental changes were needed (Blendon *et al.* 2002). In the UK, long waiting times for elective treatment were an important cause of dissatisfaction. In countries where individuals contribute to the costs of medical care, access problems were more likely to result from financial constraints. In the United States, more than half of people on below average incomes reported difficulty getting specialist treatment, having problems paying medical bills, or failing to take up tests or prescribed treatment because of cost. In all of the countries, difficulties were reported in accessing care at nights or on weekends and in obtaining dental care.

That concerns with access to health care are so widespread in countries with some of the most highly developed health services makes it relevant to explore the problems of access in more depth. This book does this from a range of disciplinary perspectives. But first we consider what is meant by 'access to health care'. The following section summarises present understanding of the term, and suggests that four main aspects should be considered.

Meaning of access

In one of the early discussions of access, Aday and Andersen (1975) suggested that 'it is perhaps most meaningful to consider access in terms of whether those who need care get into the system or not' (p. 14). They suggested that 'access' might describe either the potential or actual entry of a given individual or population group into the health care delivery system. Thus having access denotes a potential to utilise a service if required (service availability), while gaining access refers to the initiation into the process of utilising a service. Much confusion has resulted from lack of attention to these two distinct uses of the term.

Service availability

Having access to health care requires that there is an adequate supply of health services available to a population. According to this dimension, access to health care is concerned with the opportunity to obtain health care when it is wanted or needed. The availability of services is measured traditionally using indicators such as the numbers of doctors or hospital beds per unit population. In most countries there are wide geographical variations in the numbers of general practitioners per head of population, the proportion of the population registered with dentists, or the proportion accessing specialist surgical services (Department of Health 2001). These variations raise questions about the level of resources required for health care, the methods used to allocate resources to different geographical areas, and the ways that services should be configured at regional and local levels in order to optimise the availability of both primary and specialist services (see Chapter 2).

Mooney (1983) suggested that, from a health economic perspective, the availability of services may be measured in terms of the costs to individuals of obtaining care. These costs might include the costs of travel and other inconvenience incurred in obtaining care, or the health benefits forgone by not obtaining care. When services are geographically distant, these costs will be generally higher. In this formulation, individuals facing equal costs have equal access. Mooney (1983) argued that 'access is wholly a question of supply; utilisation is a function of both supply and demand' (p. 182). He went on 'It is important to stress that equality of access is about equal opportunity: the question of whether or not the opportunity is exercised is not relevant to equity defined in terms of access.'

Utilisation of services and barriers to access

Service availability can be viewed as a rather limited measure of access to health care. A population group in need may often have access to services and yet encounter difficulties in utilising services. In other words, potential access may not be realised (Aday and Anderson 1981). Thus Donabedian observed that 'the proof of access is use of service, not simply the presence of a facility' (Donabedian 1972: 111). Pechansky and Thomas (1981) developed this idea and suggested that the concept of 'access' described the 'degree of fit' between clients and the health system. The 'degree of fit' might be influenced by the acceptability, affordability and accommodation of services. Pechansky and Thomas' approach extended the concept of 'access' beyond measuring service availability, to consider the personal, organisational and financial barriers to service utilisation (Millman 1993).

Barriers to utilisation depend on the interaction of factors associated with the production of health care, such as the location of services, and factors associated with the consumption of health care, such as the ability to travel to obtain care. The value-laden term 'barrier' reflects the consumer's perception of obstacles to gaining access, and it is true that services may often be organised in a way that presents unintended obstacles to gaining access. However, from the perspective of the policy maker or service provider, methods for regulating or rationing the use of services will be required to meet financial constraints, or to achieve the equity or efficiency goals of the health service. This may result in waiting lists and other 'barriers' to care as one of a number of mechanisms for reconciling supply and demand in a publicly funded system. This again raises questions concerning how health care should be distributed: who should take the necessary decisions, and on what basis?

Personal barriers

Patients' recognition of their needs for services, and their decisions to seek medical care, generally form the first step in the process of accessing services. The probability of utilising services depends on the balance between individuals' perceptions of their needs, and their attitudes, beliefs and previous experiences with health services (Mechanic 1978). Access to health services implies that individuals identify a need for services and are willing to become service users. These perceptions of processes of access are subject to social and cultural influences as well as environmental constraints (see Chapter 4).

Individuals' expectations as service users may not always be consistent with those of health care professionals. This is evident in non-uptake of preventive services, or delays in patients presenting with serious conditions requiring treatment, or in apparently 'inappropriate' demands on general practitioners and emergency services. Policy responses have shifted in recent years from attempting to change patients' behaviours to acknowledging patients' perceptions of their needs, and managing their demands by developing a graduated service to reduce demands on general practitioners and on hospital staff in accident and emergency departments. For example, recent initiatives envisage an increased role for community pharmacies, telephone advice lines, web pages or walk-in clinics as additional pathways to access that will allow patients' concerns about less serious conditions to be addressed. Some of these developments extend the concept of access beyond the notion of physical accessibility of services, to include remote access through electronic media.

Organisational barriers

Long waiting lists and waiting times at different levels of the health care system may sometimes be indicative of organisational barriers to access which may result from a lack of capacity, an inefficient use of existing capacity, or a failure to design services around the needs of patients. Systematic variations in referral practices also act as barriers to accessing different levels of care, especially at the primary–secondary interface. The redesign of clinical service delivery methods, such as the replacement of waiting lists with booking systems, has the potential to reduce organisational barriers both to initial access to the health system and to different levels of care within the system (see Chapter 5).

Financial barriers

Financial barriers may exist at several levels and can influence the availability and utilisation of services. The overall level of resources committed to health care, and their distribution to different geographical areas and to different types of service, have a large role in determining the availability of services. Health care systems rarely use market forces as the primary method for distributing health care. There is then usually a problem that the 'supply of health care is constrained by considerations of cost, but the demand for health care will not be so constrained by consideration of price' (Klein *et al.* 1996: 9). The term 'rationing' has been used to describe the methods used to allocate resources when they are not distributed according to price (Parker 1975). Rationing may occur at the level of resource allocation, where priority-setting decisions are made, or at the level of service delivery where service providers decide who should receive a service (Klein *et al.* 1996). Both types of decision have the effect of restricting access to health care. Decision-making processes here are controversial but increasingly are being made more explicit (Chapter 11).

The payment methods used in a health care system can influence the supply of services through the incentives they offer to service providers. The demand for services will also be modified if service users make copayments for services. The UK system is mostly free at the point of use but there are charges for specific services including eye tests, dental check ups, and dispensing of prescription medicines. Other systems vary in the use of charges and other payments methods (see Chapters 6, 7 and 8). As we noted earlier, patients may also experience costs as a result of time lost from work, or in travelling to and from a clinic. The impact of user charges, and other costs of accessing care, affect different socio-economic groups in different ways. For some groups access may not be compromised, while for others costs may represent a significant deterrent (Lundberg *et al.* 1998). The impact depends on the magnitude of the costs and on the user's willingness and ability to pay. In other words, equal costs do not necessarily give equal access.

Relevance, effectiveness and access

The processes of entry into and utilisation of health care services represent only a limited part of the interaction between supply and demand for health care. The ultimate objective is to promote or preserve health. Rogers *et al.* (1999) defined optimal access as 'providing the right service at the right time in the right place'. The US Institute of Medicine defined access as the 'timely use of personal health services to achieve the best possible outcome' (Millman, 1993). These concepts introduce notions of the right service or the best possible outcomes. On this dimension, access could be measured using appropriate indicators of health status. For example, organisational barriers to access may result in delays in treatment, which can cause dissatisfaction among users and may lead to worsening clinical and patient outcomes. As the Institute of Medicine report points out, poor quality and ineffective services may be associated with high levels of utilisation but achieve unfavourable outcomes in terms of health status (Millman 1993).

Equity and access

A concern to ensure that health care resources are mobilised to meet the needs of different groups in the population is central to the concept of access. Equity introduces the notion of fairness or social justice. One of the more widely applied, and documented, definitions of equity concerns fairness in access for groups with equivalent needs. This horizontal form of equity may be evaluated with respect to health service availability, health service utilisation or health care outcomes (Mooney 1983). Most work has focused on utilisation as the preferred indicator of access, with the relationship between utilisation and need being expressed in the form of use–needs ratios, or by standardising utilisation measures for differences in needs using regression methods (Mooney 1983; van Doorslaer *et al.* 2000). The more sophisticated analyses have shown, perhaps surprisingly, little evidence of horizontal inequity in utilisation of care, even in countries where access care is considered to be severely rationed according to income (van Doorslaer *et al.* 2002). On the other hand, inequity in service availability or health outcomes has been more readily demonstrated (Chapter 3).

Another difficulty in the assessment of equity of access is that the health problems of different groups are diverse, health care needs for similar health problems vary, and different groups have their own priorities and values. Groups with different needs require access to services which are appropriately differentiated in terms of volume and quality. This vertical dimension to equity (the unequal treatment of unequals) is acknowledged to be more difficult to measure than the horizontal, not least because there is little consensus on how vertical equity could be judged to exist (Mooney 1996).

There may be an apparent tension between different objectives. Thus the desire for a universal, standard service with equality of access may conflict with the development of services based on local needs and priorities which will inevitably lead to local variations in access. This is recognised in UK policy documents which refer to the need to 'tackle the unacceptable variations that exist' while at the same time recommending that 'local doctors and nurses who ... know what patients need will be in the driving seat in shaping services' (NHS Executive 2001: 3). A key issue for those responsible for designing services is to reconcile such tensions between competing objectives, so as to facilitate appropriate utilisation of care, while at the same time safeguarding equity in treatment outcomes.

Quality of care and access

The first three proposed dimensions of access to health care correspond closely with Donabedian's three dimensions of quality of care: structure, process and outcome (Donabedian 1966). This draws attention to the relationship between access and quality of care. Maxwell (1984) identified 'accessibility' as one aspect of quality in health care, but here we have identified quality as an aspect of access. Both 'access' and 'quality' in health care are complex concepts which must be measured on several, sometimes overlapping, dimensions. However, concerns for quality and access differ in important respects. In general, quality assurance focuses attention on improving the technical and interpersonal content of individual contacts with health care services. This draws attention to the clinical effectiveness and cost-effectiveness of treatment delivered to individual patients and therefore to efficiency. By contrast, access to health care is more concerned with how health care is distributed in a population and with inequality and inequity.

Focus of the book

'Access to health care' may be understood at several levels. Following from the Covenant on Economic, Social and Cultural Rights (Office of the High Commissioner for Human Rights 1996), facilitating 'access' is concerned with helping individuals to command appropriate health care resources to preserve or improve their health. For those concerned with the organisation and delivery of health services, 'access' concerns the appropriate combination and deployment of resources to facilitate the processes of entering, and moving through the health system, in order to obtain the types of care needed to achieve optimal health outcomes. From the perspective of health policy, questions of 'access' concern the processes through which health care is distributed to those who need it, or who can pay for it.

This book explores the meaning and processes of 'access' to health care using the structure which we have set out in this introduction. The emphasis is on examining issues of access from a range of disciplinary perspectives with their focus on different levels of access and barriers to care. Chapter 2 takes a geographical approach and considers accessibility in relation to the availability of services and individuals' ability to travel for health care. Chapter 3 considers in more detail what is meant by equity and how it may be measured. It then discusses socio-economic inequalities and inequities as the main focus of attempts to achieve equity of access. Chapter 4 considers why people access services when they do not fulfil professional definitions of need, and conversely why they may not access services when they have medical needs. Chapter 5 describes organisational problems which can present barriers to access both at the level of entry into the health care system, and to patients' progress between different levels and models of care. This subject is currently the focus of much service development activity within the UK National Health Service, but the evidence for the effectiveness of different innovations is often limited. Chapter 6 discusses financial barriers to health care in terms of the overall resources available for health care, and the principles used in setting priorities, allocating resources to different types of services, and rationing the delivery of services. The chapter also considers the incentives and barriers to access offered by different methods of paying for health care services. Earlier chapters are concerned particularly with the perspective of access and policies to improve access in the UK. Chapters 7 and 8 offer contrasting views of the health systems of the United States and the countries of the European Union respectively. Important differences in approach are identified, both with respect to the extent to which universal access is identified as an objective, and in the extent to which personal financial barriers impede access to care. Chapter 9 considers these same problems as they apply to the dental service in the United Kingdom. Chapter 10 considers different approaches to the evaluation of access to health care. Finally, in the concluding chapter we return to some of the questions which have been raised in this chapter, but which remain unanswered. These concern the amount and types of health care that should be available, and how their utilisation should be regulated.

The book does not aim to be comprehensive. In particular it focuses exclusively on access to health care in the context of affluent countries, although many of the issues addressed are also of increasing concern for less affluent countries. We have deliberately not attempted to focus on specific medical problems or services, such as long-term care, mental health services or services for disabled people or carers, nor to provide detailed coverage of the specific problems for different groups of the population such as elderly people or ethnic minorities, as these issues have been reviewed elsewhere (for example Goddard and Smith 1998; Atkinson *et al.* 2001).

Note

1   Based on Gulliford, M., Figueroa-Muñoz, J., Morgan, M. *et al.* (2002) 'What does "access to health care" mean?', *J. Health Services Research Policy*, 7: 186–8.

References

Acheson, E.D. (1998) *Independent Inquiry into Inequalities in Health*. London: The Stationery Office.

Aday, L.A. and Andersen, R. (1975) *Development of Indices of Access to Medical Care*. Ann Arbor: Health Administration Press.

Aday, L.A and Anderson, R.M. (1981) 'Equity of access to medical care: a conceptual and empirical overview', *Medical Care*, 19 supplement: 4–27.

Atkinson, M., Clark, M., Clay, D., Johnson, M., Owen, D. and Szczepura, A. (2001) *Systematic Review of Ethnicity and Health Service Access for London*. Warwick: Centre for Health Services Research (University of Warwick), Mary Seacole Research Centre (de Montfort University), Centre for Research in Ethnic Relations (University of Warwick).

Blendon, R.J., Schoen, C., DesRoches, C.M., Osborn, R., Scoles, K.L. and Zapert, K. (2002) 'Inequities in health care: a five country survey', *Health Affairs*, 21: 182–91.

Bunker, J.P., Frazier, H.S. and Mosteller, F. (1994) 'Improving health: measuring effects of medical care', *The Milbank Quarterly*, 72: 225–58.

Daniels, N. (1985) *Just Health Care*. New York: Cambridge University Press.

Davidoff, F. and Reinecke, R.D. (1999) 'The 28th Amendment', *Annals of Internal Medicine*, 130: 692–4.

Deakin, N. (1994) *The Politics of Welfare: Continuities and Change*, second edition. London: Harvester Wheatsheaf.

Department of Health (2001) *High level Performance Indicators*. London: Department of Health.

Donabedian, A. (1966) 'Evaluating the quality of medical care', *Millbank Memorial Fund Quarterly*, 44 supplement: 166–206.

Donabedian, A. (1972) 'Models for organising the delivery of personal health services and criteria for evaluating them', *Milbank Memorial Fund Quarterly*, 50: 103–54.

Dworkin, R. (1977) *Taking Rights Seriously*. London: Duckworth.

Goddard, M. and Smith, P. (1998) *Equity of Access to Health Care*. York: University of York.

Hornberger, J.G. (2000) 'There is no right to health care', Future of Freedom Foundation. http://www.fff.org/comment/ed1000c.asp; accessed 21 August 2002.

Klein, R., Day, P. and Redmayne, S. (1996) *Managing Scarcity. Priority Setting and Rationing in the NHS*. Buckingham: Open University Press.

Lundberg, L., Johannesson, M., Dag, I. and Borgquist, L. (1998) 'Effects of user charges on the use of prescription medicines in different socioeconomic groups', *Health Policy*, 44: 123–34.

Maxwell, K., Streetly, A. and Bevan, D. (1999) 'Experiences of hospital care and treatment seeking for pain from sickle cell disease: qualitative study', *British Medical Journal*, 318: 1585–90.

Maxwell, R.J. (1984) 'Quality assessment in health', *British Medical Journal*, 288: 1470–2.

Mechanic, D. (1978) 'Illness behaviour'. In *Medical Sociology. A Comprehensive Text*, second edition, pp. 249–89. New York: The Free Press.

Millman, M.L. (1993) *Access to Health Care in America*. Washington, DC: Institute of Medicine, National Academy Press.

Mooney, G.H. (1983) 'Equity in health care: confronting the confusion', *Effective Health Care*, 1: 179–85.

Mooney, G.H. (1996) 'And now for vertical equity? Some concerns arising from aboriginal health in Australia', *Health Economics,* 5: 99–103.

NHS Executive (2001) *The New NHS Modern and Dependable: A National Framework for Assessing Performance*. Consultation document, Leeds: NHS Executive.

Office of the High Commissioner for Human Rights (1996) 'International Covenant on economic, social and cultural rights' Geneva: Office of the High Commissioner for Human Rights http://www.unhchr.ch/html/menu3/b/a_cescr.htm; accessed 21 August 2002.

Parker, R.A. (1975) 'Social administration and scarcity'. In E. Butterworth and R. Holman R. (eds) *Social Welfare in Modern Britain*. Glasgow: Collins Fontana.

Pechansky, R. and Thomas, W. (1981) 'The concept of access', *Medical Care*, 19: 127–40.

President's Commission for the Study of Ethical Problems in Medicine and Biomedical and Behavioural Research (1983) *Securing Access to Health Care*. Washington, DC: US Government Printing Office.

Rogers, A., Flowers, J. and Pencheon, D. (1999) 'Improving access needs a whole systems approach. And will be important in averting crises in the millenium winter', *British Medical Journal*, 319: 866–7.

Thomson, S.M.S., Pitman, D., and Mossialos, E. (2001) 'Clinical practice and the UK Human Rights Act 1998: protecting individual rights in the interests of the wider community', *Clinical Medicine*, 1: 464–9.

United Nations (1948) 'Universal declaration of human rights'. New York: United Nations. http://www.un.org.overview/rights.html; accessed 21 August 2002.

van Doorslaer, E., Wagstaff, A., van der Burg, H., Christiansen, T., De Graeve, D., Duchesne, I., Gerdtham, U.G., Gerfin, M., Geurts, J., Gross, L., Hakkinen, U., John, J., Klavus, J., Leu, R.E., Nolan, B., O'Donnell, O., Peopper, C., Puffer, F., Schellhorn, M., Sundberg, G. and Winkelhake, O. (2000) 'Equity in the delivery of health care in Europe and the US', *Journal of Health Economics*, 19: 553–83.

van Doorslaer, E., Koolman X. and Puffer F. (2002) 'Equity in the use of physician visits in OECD countries: has equal treatment for equal need been achieved?'. In P. Smith (ed) *Measuring up: Improving Health System Performance in OECD Countries* pp. 225–48. Paris: Organisation for Economic Co-operation and Development.

World Bank (1993) *World Development Report 1993*. Oxford: Oxford University Press, 1993.

Chapter 2

Geographical access to health care

Robin Haynes

Introduction

Providing equal access to health care wherever people live is not possible in most parts of the world. It is easy to demonstrate that access to health care depends on location in low-income countries, where health services are scarce, and in more developed countries where settlement is spread thinly over vast areas, as in interior parts of North America or Australia. In economically developed and densely populated regions of the Western world, however, distances to high-quality services are comparatively short and the influence of geography on access is not so obvious. This chapter examines the evidence mostly in the context of the United Kingdom, a country which has aimed to achieve geographically-uniform standards of health care for over 50 years.

'Accessibility' is the term geographers and planners use to describe the ease or difficulty of reaching services in another place. It has two main components. One is the location of services relative to the population: accessibility is high when people live close to services. The second is personal mobility, the means of reaching the destination. Services are more accessible to people who have cars than to people who do not, and where they can be reached by public transport compared to where they cannot. In an equitable world, accessibility should reflect need. People with the greatest need for a service should be able to reach it more easily than people with lesser needs.

The factors that determine geographical accessibility to health services and the consequences of variations in accessibility are summarised in Figure 2.1, which maps the structure of this chapter. In the United Kingdom, the location of health services has been determined by two opposing forces acting on the historical pattern of service availability. On the one hand, various government policies have aimed to match services to need more closely, shifting resources to places whose populations have high levels of need. On the other, a drive to make the most of scarce resources by improving efficiency and effectiveness has produced a gradual concentration of services, moving facilities to central places further from peripheral populations. Although health services are now more accessible to those in need than formerly, particularly in the poorer parts of cities, the forces of concentration

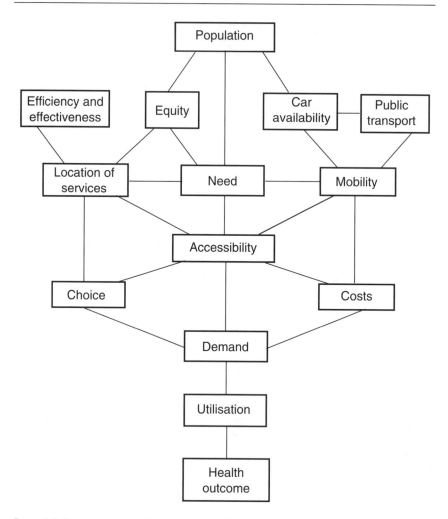

Figure 2.1 Determinants and consequences of geographical access to health care

have reduced the availability of primary and secondary care in rural districts. For most people, accessibility has not deteriorated substantially because cars have become very commonly available. At the same time, however, rural public transport services have declined and people without car transport have become more at a disadvantage. These people tend to be children, the elderly, women not in paid employment, the poor and the disabled. Perversely, the groups most in need of health care in rural Britain are those least able to reach it.

Accessibility influences the choice of services available and the costs, both monetary and non-monetary, that consumers must pay to gain access. Together these factors contribute to determining which needs for health care become demands. Variations in accessibility feed through into variations in the uptake of both primary health care and secondary hospital services. People who can easily reach health services tend to use them more than people further away. But does accessibility affect health? The evidence suggests that some health outcomes are worse than average where accessibility is poor. Geographical accessibility is one way in which health services are rationed, and the consequences are measurable. Reducing the undesirable effects will require co-ordinated efforts to reverse some longstanding trends.

Towards geographical equity

Health has a distinctive geographical pattern in the United Kingdom that reflects the distribution of wealth and poverty. People in the south enjoy generally better health than those living in the north (OPCS 1990). There is also an urban–rural gradient, with the highest morbidity and mortality rates in the large cities and lower rates in rural areas (Phillimore and Reading 1992; Haynes and Gale 1999; Senior et al. 2000).

Before the foundation of the National Health Service in 1946, the availability of health services in the UK was determined not by the needs but by the income levels of local communities. The resulting distribution was described later as the 'inverse care law': the availability of good medical care tends to vary inversely with the need of the population served (Hart 1971). One of the main aims of the new national service was to ensure that 'an equally good service is available everywhere' (Bevan 1945), but disparities in the quality and quantity of health services between places were reduced only slowly. The inverse care law still applies in many parts of the country. For example, there are 50 per cent more general practitioners in parts of affluent south east England compared with some industrial towns in northern England after adjusting for age and health care needs (Department of Health 2000a).

Much has been achieved by gradually directing resources to the areas with greatest need. Redistribution of general practitioners from the more affluent areas to the less attractive districts, often low-income communities in the inner cities, was an early priority. The Medical Practices Committee was introduced to control the geographical distribution of medical practitioners, with powers to refuse an application to practise in a certain place if it considered that the number of doctors relative to the number of patients there was adequate (Medical Practices Committee 2000). Now the task is incorporated into a national formula for allocating resources (Department of Health 2000a).

In the early years of the NHS, central funding was allocated to maintain existing services, but a succession of government policies to reduce geographical inequities in the availability of hospital and community services through formula funding began with the report of the Resource Allocation Working Party in England (DHSS 1976). The report recommended that resources should be distributed on the basis of the size of the population adjusted according to the local needs for health care (based on the general level of health) and unavoidable differences in the cost of staff salaries, building and land from place to place. The immediate effect was to suggest that the south east had been over-funded relative to other parts of England. In order to dampen sudden changes in financial provision, health authorities were gradually moved year by year towards their target positions. The same principles still apply, and to other parts of the UK, although the measurement of additional needs for health care has become more sophisticated. At first, the formulae used standardised mortality ratios, but later versions have added census information in composite measures of need (Department of Health 1999b). Examples of the census information include the prevalence of limiting long-term illness, the unemployment rate, the proportions of elderly persons living alone and dependents in single carer households, all of which have been shown to predict small area variations in service use after removing the effects of local variations in supply (Smith *et al.* 1994).

The resource allocation method is designed to give fair shares to areas with populations of several hundred thousand – originally health authorities and now primary care trusts – and not to ensure that resources are spread equitably at the most local level. That is a matter for each commissioning authority to determine. It makes no attempt to make up for any deficiencies in housing, environmental quality or social services provision. Treating the health service as an independent entity is most likely to disadvantage inner city communities, whose demands on the health services are increased by worse conditions in other respects. On the other hand, measuring needs indirectly through use and not directly through morbidity might introduce systematic bias to the detriment of rural populations with lower utilisation rates (Asthana *et al.* 2002). The method does recognise higher salary and building costs in achieving the same level of service relative to need in London and other metropolitan areas compared with the national average, but does not take any possible rural premiums into account (Woollett 1990). Higher costs in rural areas might be expected from the lack of economies of scale, the additional costs of travel, additional telecommunication costs, the unproductive time spent in travelling, the extra costs of providing outreach services and the extra costs of accessing training and other support (Watt and Sheldon 1993; Asthana *et al.* 2002). These higher unit costs are acknowledged in some situations. General practitioners receive an allowance based on their patients' distance from the surgery and in Scotland and Wales, but not in England, the resource allocation formulae include a small weighting for the effects of population sparsity on providing community health services. There is no allowance for any rural premium for hospital services in England, an omission that is inconsistent (Watt and Sheldon 1993).

Not only the quantity but also the quality of primary care services has a geographical expression in the UK. Access to high-quality primary care is at its worst in decaying parts of inner cities, the very places where health is poorest (London Health Planning Consortium 1981; Tomlinson 1992). Reforms were introduced in 1990 with a new contract for general practitioners, and from then general practitioners working in 'underprivileged areas' were paid more money, based on the argument that demands on them are greater than on doctors elsewhere. Underprivileged areas are identified from a weighted combination of population census variables based on patient characteristics that a national sample of general practitioners said affected their workload (Jarman 1983; Martin *et al.* 1994). Spurred by unmistakable evidence that poverty produces illness (DHSS 1980; Acheson 1998), the most recent policies for socially deprived areas have concentrated on broader local initiatives to improve health by reducing social exclusion. These include the New Deal programme to regenerate the most deprived neighbourhoods by improving economic and employment opportunities, the Sure Start programme which promotes the health and wellbeing of pre-school children and Health Action Zones, where better co-ordinated and seamless services are being encouraged (Department of Health 1999a).

Centralisation of services

The policies described so far were intended to make services more equitably available from place to place. At the same time, pressures to increase efficiency and effectiveness within the National Health Service have worked in another direction, draining services from outlying locations and concentrating them in central places. In primary care, single practising doctors used to be the norm, but are now a rarity. Compared with only 2,000 single-handed practices there are now over 8,000 doctors in practices with six or more partners (Medical Practices Committee 2000). The growth of large partnerships brought professional and financial benefits to GPs. The geographical effect was a concentration of primary care into larger, fewer and more dispersed surgeries. In the cities and towns patients were little affected, but rural communities noticed the difference. Surgeries in outlying villages were closed, to be replaced by an enlarged group practice surgery in the largest village or small town, serving what was formerly the territory of several practices. Some rural practices still maintain more than one surgery, but many branch surgeries with simple facilities and restricted opening hours have gone. Home visiting rates declined at the same time (Cartwright and Anderson 1981; Whewell *et al.* 1983). The result was an increase in the average distance people had to travel to see their doctor.

The geographical pattern of hospital services in the UK has also been changing. While monolithic psychiatric hospitals have been replaced by dispersed community services, non-psychiatric hospitals have become much more concentrated. Fifty years ago, hospitals varied enormously in size, function and physical condition. The Hospital Plan first set out the objective: a network of large district general hospitals, each providing specialised medical and surgical facilities for a catchment of 200,000 to 300,000 population (Ministry of Health 1962). All district general hospitals were based in the larger centres of population. Later policies relating to particular hospital services, such as accident and emergency departments, maternity services and operating departments endorsed the advantages of large units in terms of the organisation of work, staffing arrangements, career structures, the cost of technological equipment and better outcomes for patients. Over the years, general hospitals were either extended vertically on inner city sites or relocated to greenfield sites on the fringes of cities. Many small hospitals were closed, usually in the face of local public opposition.

Scientific advances in treatment continue to favour more concentration. Cancer patients treated in specialist facilities, for example, receive more up to date treatment, and have lower peri-operative mortality rates, fewer recurrences and improved chances of survival (Campbell *et al.* 1999). Typical district general hospitals are now encouraged to limit their contribution to the routine treatment of common cancers, and specialist diagnostic and therapeutic services for cancer have been further concentrated in selected centres (Department of Health 2000b). Policies to improve the effectiveness of acute hospital services have almost invariably made them more distant for people living outside the main towns and cities.

The efficiency argument was, perhaps, overplayed. Some critics have questioned the quality of evidence that has been used to justify policies of increasing concentration of health services into ever-larger units. Studies that claimed to show that greater volume produces better health outcomes often did not control sufficiently for complications such as differences in case mix, and did not establish the direction of causality (Sowden *et al.* 1997). Economies of scale for acute general hospitals become exhausted between 200 and 400 beds; above this size, unit costs are probably higher (Aletras *et al.* 1997). Larger units are not necessarily more efficient or more effective according to this view.

Transport and mobility

Two long-term trends have had a substantial effect on the ability of people to reach health services in the United Kingdom. The ownership and availability of private car transport has steadily risen, while public transport has declined. These trends have occurred most distinctly in rural areas. Rural households are more likely to have access to a car (87 per cent) than urban households (78 per cent) and also tend to have more vehicles (Countryside Agency 2001b). For rural populations, private transport is often a precondition for employment and a necessity for accessing other essential services (Shucksmith *et al.* 1996). Rural populations in the UK on average tend to be more affluent than people living in cities, but averages hide considerable variations. About one quarter of households in rural areas live in or close to the borders of poverty (McLaughlin 1986; Cloke *et al.* 1995; Cox 1998). Households with low incomes in rural areas have to make sacrifices in order to run a car. Some low-income and elderly households have no car, and some members of one-car households rarely have the use of it, typically because it is dedicated to one person's journey to work. The least mobile groups are children and teenagers, the elderly and women not in employment and not in two-car households. In addition, and overlapping, are the poor and disabled (Moseley 1979). Collectively these people comprise a substantial proportion of the rural population. They are the groups with the highest needs for health care.

Public transport services are still relatively good in most urban areas, but regular bus services have disappeared from many country districts. Only 51 per cent of rural settlements have a bus service for six or seven days a week and 29 per cent of all rural settlements have no bus service (Countryside Agency 2001a). Policies to reduce the problems of social exclusion arising from poor accessibility to essential services in rural areas were highlighted in the Rural White Paper (Department for Environment Food and Rural Affairs 2000). Since 1997, significant improvements in rural transport have been funded by government.

Measures of accessibility based on distance and time

Personal mobility is crucial in determining whether or not services can be reached, but most measures of geographical accessibility concentrate on the physical separation that impedes contact. Impedance (the 'friction of distance') can be represented by straight line distance, distance along the road network, travel time or travel cost. Of these, straight line distance is easiest to compute and is generally highly correlated with the other measures (Phibbs and Luft 1995). Road distance, time or cost are more direct measures of impedance levels actually experienced, particularly in regions with a patchy road network, physical barriers such as major rivers or hills, or an irregular coastline (Martin *et al.* 2002). Variations in the use of health services are more strongly associated with road distance and estimated travel time than with straight line distance (Martin *et al.* 1998).

The average distance from a community to the nearest service is a common measure (Higgs and White 2000). The location of a community is approximated as a single point at the population-weighted centre ('centroid') of a small administrative area. This point and the service location given by its postcode are represented as co-ordinates on the national grid, and straight line distances between them are calculated from Pythagoras's theorem. Using this method the Countryside Agency (2001a) found that 86 per cent of all households in England live within 4 km of a doctor's surgery and 92 per cent of households in rural areas live within 12 km of a hospital.

Alternatively, the road distance or travel time by car can be estimated, typically in a geographic information system or GIS (Longley *et al.* 2001). In such studies, the GIS is used to find the nearest service from each population location along the road network, then the distances along road segments are added to produce the total road distance. A refinement is to use the road class and average speeds on various classes of road to estimate average car travel times from population locations to services. In Cambridgeshire, Norfolk and Suffolk, for example, 67 per cent of the population was estimated to be less than 5 minutes by car from a GP surgery but 10 per cent of the population lived more than 10 minutes from a surgery (Lovett *et al.* 2002).

The nearest service is not necessarily the one that is actually used. Perhaps about half of GP registrations are with the nearest practice (Salisbury 1989; Lovett *et al.* 2000), so measures of access to primary health care based on the nearest surgery typically underestimate the journeys that are actually made (Martin and Williams 1992). Measures of the level of choice available at any location must recognise that increasing distance, cost or travel time makes each destination progressively less attractive. For any consumer, the available choice of surgeries, for instance, can be summarised by counting the total number of surgeries, each weighted by how far away it is, so that distant surgeries have very little influence compared with opportunities nearby. The impedance weighting may have various mathematical forms. The resulting measure of accessibility to all services is termed the 'potential' (Joseph and Bantock 1982; Martin and Williams 1992; Higgs and White 2000).

Distances or travel times by car are sometimes incorporated into evaluations of alternative patterns of service provision, particularly hospital location strategies. One approach compares alternative locations by measuring the distance or travel time from all population centres (typically, census area centroids) to the nearest services in question, expressing the results as the average travel distance or maps of travel times (Lovett et al. 1998). This method can incorporate different levels of need indicated by variations in population characteristics, but it assumes that demand is not affected by accessibility. An alternative, known as 'spatial interaction' or 'gravity' modelling, takes the diminution in demand with increased distance (or travel time) observed under current circumstances as a starting point, and builds a 'distance decay' of trips into future location scenarios. Tacket's (1989) evaluation of different arrangements of inpatient facilities in East Anglia and Congdon's (2000) models of patient flows to hospital emergency services in London before and after restructuring are examples. While the first method might be accused of being idealistic, the second acknowledges, and perhaps perpetuates, an inequitable distribution of benefits.

Accessibility by public transport

It is more difficult to measure the accessibility of services by public transport. In some rural parts of Britain, bus services are less frequent than hourly and limited to certain days of the week. Bus services almost invariably go to centres of population where key services such as GP surgeries are found, so the availability of a bus service usually means that primary health care can be reached. The National Travel Survey found that 42 per cent of a sample of households in rural Britain were within 13 minutes' walk of a bus route with an hourly service (Countryside Agency 2001b). This figure does not reveal how the proportion varied from place to place. Higgs and White (2000) took a more geographical approach, assembling information on bus services from responses to a questionnaire sent to Community Councils in Wales and mapping the results. This method overestimated the availability of public transport because it did not take the dispersion of people within each community into account. Lovett et al. (2002) overcame the difficulty, using a GIS to identify postcode locations within walking distance of bus routes with varying levels of service frequency. They found that for most people in East Anglia there was a daytime bus service with at least four return trips to a surgery, but 13 per cent of the population lived in places with no return daytime service to a surgery. Further refinements incorporate bus travel times and connecting services (Martin *et al.* 2002). Such methods are computer-intensive and require much manual work with timetables, but electronic timetable systems are developing rapidly and it will soon be possible to assemble accurate time and cost information about public transport in a GIS framework (Martin *et al.* 2002).

The problem of reducing accessibility to a single average measure for a village or small census area is that it glosses over the spectrum of personal mobility. To say that a village enjoys a certain level of accessibility is to ignore the distinction between, for example, an employed adult in a two-car household and an elderly person without a car: neighbours living in different worlds (Moseley 1979). Moseley advocated a method that recognised the variations within each community, focusing on particular groups and particular activities and recognising the importance of time. If a car was available only in the evening and at weekends, or if a bus service operated only twice a week, for instance, did the local surgery open at those times? Painstaking local fieldwork rather than computing power is needed to implement this approach fully, although the concept of public transport dependency does offer a compromise. Nutley (1980) defined total and partial dependency as the proportions of people without a household car or with a share in a household car. Both measures come from routine census information. Nutley, and more recently Higgs and White (2000), found that in Wales the proportions of total dependency were low by national standards, reflecting high levels of car ownership especially in the areas with the worst public transport services.

Social benefits and costs

What differences do variations in geographical access make to people's lives? One obvious effect, neglected in the research literature, is that people with high levels of accessibility have more choice and take advantage of it. In the UK, the choice of hospital is made more commonly by general practitioners than by patients, but people are usually able to register with the general practitioner of their preference. The availability of choice depends on the distribution and density of services, and so has an urban–rural dimension. Cities have large numbers of general practices within a relatively small travel time of each other, and residents are able to exercise considerable choice. In one inner city council estate in Edinburgh, for example, 1,433 people were registered with 87 GPs in 43 practices (Murray *et al.* 1995). In rural parishes, most residents register with the nearest practice (Lovett *et al.* 2000) with, perhaps, some loss of satisfaction. Anonymity in the waiting room is not possible, for example.

Other costs are more tangible. Rural populations face higher than average costs to reach services. The health service does not consider anything other than its own direct costs, and has no incentive to do so, but decisions on the pattern of health services inevitably have implications for the costs paid by individual patients and society in general (Watt and Sheldon 1993). Consumers of health care bear not only the cost of travel but also the cost of the time involved, which might involve paid and unpaid work, childcare and leisure activities, and all these are directly related to the distance between home and service and have a disproportionate effect on the poor (Gibson *et al.* 1985). There is no shortage of anecdotal evidence of costly, difficult and painful journeys to hospital for investigation or treatment (for example Baird *et al.* 2000). Travel can also be expensive and inconvenient for visitors to hospital patients, so rural patients separated from home have a greater emotional burden. Visiting rates decline with distance and length of stay (Cross and Turner 1974; Haynes and Bentham 1979). In the most remote communities, the grief of bereavement is sharpened when a person dies unvisited in a distant hospital (Bloor *et al.* 1978).

Accessibility and utilisation

In geography, the general relationship between activity rates and accessibility is known as 'distance decay'. Almost all forms of human activity are reduced in frequency by distance or travel time (Haggett *et al.* 1977) and the use of health services is no exception. The first known record noted that people living close to an insane hospital were more likely to become patients than those living further away (Jarvis 1850). Many studies since have confirmed the pattern, although most have been cross-sectional designs poorly adjusted for the effects of variations in need (Joseph and Phillips 1984; Watt 1995; Carr-Hill *et al.* 1997).

The effect of accessibility on general practitioner consultations is of particular interest because the GP is the gatekeeper to secondary health care in the UK. The weight of evidence from different contexts suggests that decreasing consultation rates with worsening accessibility are not an artefact of uncontrolled variables, but few studies have demonstrated this directly. The fourth national study of morbidity statistics from general practice (OPCS 1995) was a very large study of consultation behaviour, covering a 1 per cent sample of the population of England and Wales. Distance from the practice was found to be generally a deterrent to consultation. A multivariate analysis of these data, which controlled for a large number of variables at the individual level together with socio-economic conditions in the place of residence, suggested that both distance to the practice and residence in a rural area exerted independent effects on rates of consultation (Carr-Hill *et al.* 1996).

The fourth national morbidity study did find that the deterrent effect of distance on consultations was stronger for less serious illnesses (OPCS 1995). Some health conditions are considered not to be serious enough for a trip to the doctor, and the doctor's accessibility probably influences the decision. Self-referral of patients to hospital accident and emergency departments shows the same characteristic. Rates of attendance at an accident and emergency department for injuries to pre-school children were progressively diminished with increasing distance. Distance had a weaker effect on attendance for more serious injuries, although it was still statistically significant (Reading *et al.* 1999).

There would be little cause for concern if only the less serious conditions were affected by distance, but reduced contacts with primary care are matched by lower use of hospital services. In Norfolk, random samples of urban and rural residents were questioned on their recent use of GP, outpatient and inpatient services, and use/needs ratios were calculated, crudely adjusting utilisation rates for morbidity variations from place to place (Bentham and Haynes 1985). The use/needs ratios were highest in the city, higher in villages with a surgery than in those without, and higher in villages close to the general hospital than in more distant villages. The ratios were also higher for people from households with a car and a telephone and lower for those without both. Use as a ratio of needs was at least three times higher for mobile people in the city compared with less mobile people in the least accessible villages, and this was found for GP consultations, outpatient attendances and inpatient episodes. How the three stages were connected could not be shown by a cross-sectional study; this would require a longitudinal design to trace the process from illness to admission.

As with primary care consultations, few research studies have been able to control for confounding variables when comparing the use of hospital facilities from place to place. This weakness is especially serious for studies of hospital utilisation because populations with high health care needs tend to be found close to hospitals in inner city locations. The most sophisticated analysis of small area variations in inpatient episodes was carried out by economists at the University of York to identify a suitable combination of measures of the need for hospital services for resource allocation purposes (Carr-Hill et al. 1994). A two-stage model was used to take into account the complex relationship between needs, supply and use. Re-examination of the data suggested to the authors that hospital episodes were affected by distance to general practitioner but not distance to hospital (Carr-Hill et al. 1997). This interpretation should be treated with caution because the original model was not designed to test the effect of distance, but to hold constant any combined effect of 'supply' factors. Supply was measured as the number of hospital beds or the number of general practitioners divided (for technical reasons) by 10 km plus distance to the service squared. The re-examination used the same composite supply measure, not a simple measure of distance.

A more direct test was made using comparable data covering the East Anglian region (Haynes et al. 1999). Ward variations between hospital episode ratios adjusted for age and sex composition were compared with all the indicators of need identified as important in the York study and with measures of provision and distance. Distance to the nearest appropriate hospital and to the nearest GP surgery was measured for each ward. Needs indicators were found to be the most important determinants of emergency acute and psychiatric inpatient variations from place to place, but variations in service provision were more important for elective acute and geriatric inpatient episodes. Hospital episodes were inversely related to both distance measures before any adjustment. Holding needs and provision measures statistically constant, distance to hospital reduced inpatient episodes of all types significantly. Distance to the nearest GP surgery had a weaker effect on hospital episodes, statistically significant for elective but not for emergency acute admissions. This distinction raised the possibility that earlier- rather than later-stage contacts with primary care had been influenced by accessibility.

When hospital services are manifestly in short supply there is clear evidence of rationing by accessibility. Several studies of renal replacement therapy and cardiac surgery illustrate the point. Renal replacement therapy is based in specialist units, and uptake is inversely related to distance to the unit (Dalziel and Garrett 1987; Will *et al.* 1987). In two districts with similar incidence of renal failure, referral of patients for renal replacement therapy was more likely in the district with a unit than in the district without a unit (Feest *et al.* 1990). Renal replacement therapy referral rates in south-west Wales, partially controlled for deprivation and ethnicity, were negatively related to distance for patients over 60 years old, but not significantly for younger groups (Boyle *et al.* 1996). Martin *et al.* (1998) analysed data on patients accepted for renal replacement therapy at all renal units in England. The results confirmed the primary importance of age, sex, ethnicity and deprivation in explaining variations in treatment rates and, with these held constant, revealed a significant effect of distance from the unit. This was interpreted as a sign that there are barriers to referral for less accessible populations. Studies of the effects of accessibility on the uptake of cardiac surgery have had similar results. In the North East Thames region there were higher rates of coronary artery bypass grafts in districts containing cardiothoracic surgical facilities than in other districts, adjusting for age and deprivation (Ben-Shlomo and Chaturvedi 1995). A second ecological study confirmed higher rates of revascularisation in English and Scottish districts close to specialist cardiology facilities than elsewhere, and found some evidence that intervention rates were inversely related to needs (Black *et al.* 1995).

Accessibility and health outcomes

Renal replacement therapy and cardiac surgery are extreme examples, because both are directly linked to survival. Variations in the use of health services do not necessarily lead to worse health outcomes, although some association might be anticipated. The evidence is discussed in relation to ambulance response times and the accessibility to hospital for asthma and cancer patients.

There is little evidence that ambulance response times in the United Kingdom substantially affect outcomes, although ambulance response is believed to be critical for some conditions. Most deaths from myocardial infarction, for example, occur outside hospital, and ambulance delays of more than 8 minutes lead to a high probability of an unfavourable outcome. Dunn *et al.* (2000) found strong regional variations in case fatality of myocardial infarction, with the lowest rates in Scotland and the highest in southern England. Ambulance delay was suggested as a plausible explanation. On the national scale, ambulance response times are not necessarily highest in the most rural districts because of traffic congestion in the major metropolitan areas. The proportion of ambulance delays of longer than 8 minutes to cardiac arrest calls at the time was highest in London, and lower in

Scotland than in England as a whole, but no further support for the hypothesis was available.

Road traffic accidents are a major cause of death for children and young adults in the United Kingdom and some places are at an apparent disadvantage in terms of the time taken by ambulances to reach an incident and get to hospital. American evidence has suggested that traffic accident victims who had to wait longest for treatment were more likely to die (Brown 1979). In England and Wales, local authority districts with no accident and emergency department had a higher mortality rate from road traffic accidents than districts with accident and emergency facilities (Bentham 1986). To avoid the problems of ecological inference, a further study used police records of individual accidents to estimate the odds of death versus serious injury in a rural county where total ambulance journey times might extend to 50 minutes (Jones and Bentham 1995). A higher probability of death was found for the elderly, pedestrians, casualties from multiple collisions and casualties on roads with higher speed limits but no relationship was found between fatality and estimated ambulance time. The authors concluded that the previous result of high mortality in remoter rural districts might have been the result of more severe accidents on fast rural roads. Ambulance response times did not appear to be a cause for concern in Norfolk.

The same authors investigated asthma deaths. Most asthma deaths are potentially preventable with timely and appropriate intervention. Using aggregate data for local authority districts in England and Wales and holding district variations in socio-economic variables constant, Jones and Bentham (1997) detected a rise in asthma mortality in proportion to the distance to the nearest large acute hospital. A delay in seeking specialist medical attention seemed the most biologically plausible explanation (Garrett 1997). A more detailed examination of asthma deaths in wards in three counties revealed a consistent tendency for asthma mortality to increase with estimated travel time to hospital (Jones *et al.* 1999). No trend with estimated time to the nearest GP surgery was apparent. A third study, based on a 10 per cent population survey of one constituent health authority, investigated the link with consultation rates (Jones *et al.* 1998). It confirmed that the likelihood of consulting a hospital doctor for breathing problems decreased with estimated travel time to hospital, but the likelihood of a GP consultation for respiratory problems was not affected by time to the nearest surgery. This suggested that for asthma sufferers the accessibility of hospital care has more serious repercussions than access to primary care. Studies from other countries confirm that distance to services influences the help-seeking behaviour of people with asthma (Garrett *et al.* 1986; Taytard *et al.* 1990) and that general practitioners are less likely to refer patients living in remote locations for specialist treatment than patients living nearer to secondary facilities (Fylkesnes *et al.* 1992).

Delays in seeking treatment have also been suggested as the explanation for raised cancer death rates in remote districts. A study of colorectal cancer registrations in Calvados, France, provided the first link between variations in the use of services and survival. Launoy *et al.* (1992) observed a gradient with accessibility in the proportion of patients of both sexes who were treated in specialised centres. For males there was no difference in survival between urban and rural populations, but women from rural residences had a lower survival rate than urban women. Controlling for age, tumour extension symptoms and type of treatment removed the urban–rural difference in survival in women, suggesting that the isolation of rural women led to delayed diagnosis, different treatment and worse survival. Other results from several countries are consistent. These have shown that people remote from specialist cancer centres are likely to present with more advanced tumours (Liff *et al.* 1991; Montella *et al.* 1995), are less likely to receive treatment with radiotherapy and chemotherapy (Greenberg *et al.* 1988; Craft *et al.* 1997) and have poorer prognoses (Bonett *et al.* 1990).

In the UK, rural GPs have complained of problems in gaining access to cancer treatment for patients living in remoter areas (Baird et. al. 2000). Campbell *et al.* (2000) investigated whether late diagnosis and survival from cancer differed for Scottish patients in rural and urban areas. Data on patients with lung, colorectal, breast, prostate, stomach and ovarian cancers were linked with information about their places of residence. The proportion of patients who were diagnosed on their date of death was used as an indicator of late diagnosis. This proportion increased significantly with distance for colorectal, breast and stomach cancers with and without adjustments for age, sex and settlement size. Apparent distance effects on survival were present for all cancer sites, and poorer survival for lung cancer and prostate cancers was significantly associated with increasing distance from a cancer centre, holding age, sex, deprivation and settlement size constant. Kim *et al.* (2000) also found post-operative survival from colorectal cancer declined with increasing distance from a treatment centre in southern England. Coinciding with the appearance of these studies, the NHS Cancer Plan set out to concentrate cancer services further, to improve survival (Department of Health 2000b). Centralisation may, indeed, save more lives overall, but not without cost.

Improving geographical access

Interventions to improve geographical access to health services might be divided into those that bring people to services, those that move services closer to people and those that reduce barriers other than distance. While promising interventions have been identified, few well-designed studies offer rigorous evaluations (Goddard and Smith 1998).

Current policies to facilitate the movement of people to services target those with no access, or limited access, to private car transport. Since 1997 government subsidies for conventional bus services have been increased substantially and the Ten Year Transport Plan has a target to increase by one third the proportion of rural households living within a 10-minute walk of an hourly service (Department of Environment Transport and the Regions 2000). For small settlements off the main road system, scheduled commercial bus services are not the solution because demand is too low and variable. Here, community transport schemes are being encouraged by government grants. Community car schemes typically involve volunteer drivers using their own cars to provide door-to door journeys for people without transport, while dial-a-ride services commonly use minibuses and may focus particularly on individuals with restricted mobility. The Rural Services Survey found that 48 per cent of rural parishes operated community transport schemes in 2000 compared with 18 per cent in 1991 (Countryside Agency 2001a). Some schemes are run by volunteers and serve an area of no more than one or two parishes, while others have a much larger scope and employ co-ordinators and drivers. There appears to be considerable variability in public awareness and usage levels between schemes, but little research on the factors that contribute towards effectiveness. While much of the responsibility for transport lies beyond the compass of the health service, more could be done from within health services to ameliorate transport difficulties. Consultation times that fit in with transport availability would help, together with block booking for clinic appointments from the same rural area to facilitate transport sharing and more efficient routing of ambulance transport.

While strong forces have acted to centralise health facilities, there are both long-established and new opportunities to bring services closer to users. In rural primary care, there is still a role for outlying consultation facilities with limited opening hours and simple facilities to encourage first contacts, at least in the transition years before communication innovations make a difference. Doctors see greater proportions of elderly patients, females, people with lower incomes and people without cars in outlying facilities than in their main surgeries, and low consultation rates in settlements with no surgery are raised by the presence of an outlying branch facility (Fearn et al. 1984). Mobile surgeries and mobile units for screening increase take-up rates and are acceptable to those attending (Haiart et al. 1990; Bentham and Haynes 1992).

Several schemes in which hospital specialists have provided outpatient clinics in general practice premises have been assessed (Roland and Shapiro 1998). It is not clear whether these schemes are cost effective (Mead et al. 1998), but they appear to perform at least as well as general hospital outpatient departments in terms of waiting times, attendance rates, and length of episode. Outreach clinics for cancer treatment, which involve specialists travelling to rural clinics and sharing care with local practitioners, appear to be safe, and might be combined with televideo links (Campbell et al. 1999). Other hospital services, such as simple day surgery, might also be extended beyond the district hospital setting. Minor surgery in small local hospitals can be as cost-effective as centralised care (Soper and Jones 1985). A day surgery service for cataract provided in a small hospital produced comparable health outcomes but was more popular with patients than the main hospital alternative 40 km away (Haynes et al. 2001). Patients appreciated the smaller scale of the outreach clinic, which made it a more friendly and supportive environment. Patients generally prefer to attend local clinics where they are available because of shorter and more convenient journeys (Bailey et al. 1994; Gillam et al. 1995; Black et al. 1997; Bowling et al. 1997).

The NHS Plan (Department of Health 2000a) has acknowledged that there is near-universal public support for the development of care closer to home, and the shift in funding from health authorities to locally based primary care trusts could help to balance the long-term trend towards centralisation. The plan includes provision for developing intermediate inpatient services between primary and secondary hospital care, some in community or cottage hospitals.

Other policy options might be directed at reducing constraints and discontinuities that hinder access for immobile groups. One possibility is for health services to become more active in making contact with hard-to-reach patients. For some people, health might at times seem unimportant and not worth the effort of a trip to the doctor. Haiart *et al.* (1990) found that uptake of opportunistic breast screening in a mobile unit was adversely affected by distance, but that personal invitations from general practitioners produced a 75 per cent response rate in women who had failed to attend previously. Similarly, Bentham *et al.* (1995) found that the uptake of opportunistic cervical cytology screening was adversely affected by remoteness, but remoteness was no longer a significant deterrent when a population-based call and recall system was introduced.

Gateways into health care services that do not involve physical transport might be developed further. Telephone consultation is becoming an increasingly accepted approach to patient care and telephone consultations with experienced and specially trained nurses have been shown to be a safe and effective means of first contact (Lattimer *et al.* 1998). NHS Direct, a 24-hour nurse-led service which provides clinical advice, general information and referral to other health services by telephone (Department of Health 1997) might benefit immobile people in less accessible locations particularly, but this has yet to be demonstrated. Telemedicine will also be beneficial. There is evidence that health services can be successfully and effectively delivered to rural areas by using telecommunications and information technologies, but almost all of it relates to work done outside the United Kingdom (Wootton 1999).

There is scope, too, for reducing the boundaries between health care professionals by broader training, so that one professional might substitute for several in places where services are thin on the ground. Nurse practitioners are increasingly acting as the point of first contact in primary care, offering high-quality care and high levels of patient satisfaction (Venning *et al.* 2000; Horrocks *et al.* 2002). Nurse clinics and enhanced home visiting by nurses might boost primary care in some areas. Better co-ordination between primary care and secondary care, and between acute hospitals and tertiary centres, is required to escape from the constraints of historical referral patterns based on links between individuals. The planned development of 'cancer networks' (Commission for Health Improvement 2001) and other clinical networks (Baker and Lorimer 2000) might in the future improve co-ordination between services and provide rural patients with a more integrated programme of care. Local initiatives adapted to local circumstances (Fearn 1987) will still have a part to play.

Conclusions

Even in a densely-populated country with highly-developed health services, it is not possible to achieve the aim of fair access to health care based on need alone, irrespective of where people live (Department of Health 1997) because the geographical separation of people and services makes inequalities inevitable. Geographical inaccessibility increases the costs of reaching health services, reduces the use made of them and, in some cases, leads to worse health. The burden falls disproportionately on the poor. What can be done is to lessen rather than remove these effects.

Little is known about the costs and effectiveness of the various intervention strategies available. Effective policies will target the mechanisms, but there is much to learn here, too. The people most affected by inaccessibility, residents of rural areas without personal transport, are difficult to find, and we have no clear idea of the relative significance of barriers to be overcome before the first contact with health services and at the various stages of care from then on. A longitudinal study of immobile people in a rural setting, tracing the sequence from lifestyle to illness to outcome through the stages of health care, would fill some of the gaps in current knowledge.

Health service planners should begin to acknowledge that policies to improve medical outcome and make best use of internal resources incur social costs outside the health care system. Trade-offs are made, choosing gains in cost, efficiency or effectiveness at the expense of a loss in geographical accessibility, and these decisions are often taken without being acknowledged. Implicit judgements of this sort should be aired and the consequences considered. Reducing the rationing of health care by geographical accessibility will require resources, so the priority of this aim relative to others deserves wider public debate.

References

Acheson, D. (Chairman) (1998) *Independent Inquiry into Inequalities in Health: Report.* London: The Stationery Office.

Aletras, V., Jones, A. and Sheldon, T.A. (1997) 'Economies of scale and scope'. In B. Ferguson, T. Sheldon and J. Posnett (eds) *Concentration and Choice in Healthcare.* London: Financial Times Healthcare.

Asthana, S., Brigham, P. and Gibson, A. (2002) *Health Resource Allocation in England: What Case Can be Made for Rurality?* Plymouth: University of Plymouth.

Bailey, J.J., Black, M.E. and Wilkin, D. (1994) 'Specialist outreach clinics in general practice', *British Medical Journal*, 308: 1083–6.

Baird, A.G., Donnelly, C.M., Miscampell, N.T. and Wemyss, H.D. (2000) 'Centralisation of cancer services in rural areas has disadvantages', *British Medical Journal*, 320: 717.

Baker, C.D. and Lorimer, A.R. (2000) 'Cardiology: the development of a managed clinical network', *British Medical Journal*, 321: 1152–3.

Ben-Shlomo, Y. and Chaturvedi, N. (1995) 'Assessing equity in access to health care provision in the UK: does where you live affect your chances of getting a coronary artery bypass graft?', *Journal of Epidemiology and Community Health*, 49: 200–4.

Bentham, G. (1986) 'Proximity to hospital and mortality from motor vehicle traffic accidents', *Social Science and Medicine*, 23: 1021–6.

Bentham, G. and Haynes, R. (1985) 'Health, personal mobility and the use of health services in rural Norfolk', *Journal of Rural Studies*, 1: 231–9.

Bentham, G. and Haynes, R. (1992) 'Evaluation of a mobile branch surgery in a rural area', *Social Science and Medicine*, 34: 97–102.

Bentham, G., Hinton, J., Haynes, R., Lovett, A. and Bestwick, C. (1995) 'Factors affecting non-response to cervical cytology screening in Norfolk, England', *Social Science and Medicine*, 40: 131–5.

Bevan, A. (1945) *Memorandum by the Minister of Health to the Cabinet*, 5 October 1945, CAB 129/3. London: Public Record Office.

Black, M., Leese, B., Gosden, T. and Mead, N. (1997) 'Specialists' outreach clinics in general practice: what do they offer?', *British Journal of General Practice*, 47: 558–61.

Black, N., Langham, S. and Petticrew, M. (1995) 'Coronary revascularisation: why do rates vary geographically in the UK?', *Journal of Epidemiology and Community Health*, 49: 408–12.

Bloor, M., Horobin, G., Taylor, R. and Williams, R. (1978) *Island Health Care: Access to Primary Services in the Western Isles*, Occasional Paper 3. Aberdeen: Institute of Sociology, University of Aberdeen.

Bonett, A., Dorsch, M., Roder, D., Esterman, A. (1990) 'Infiltrating ductal carcinoma of the breast in South Australia', *Medical Journal of Australia*, 152: 19–23.

Bowling, A., Stramer, K., Dickinson, E., Windsor, J. and Bond, M. (1997) 'Evaluation of specialists' outreach clinics in general practice in England: process and acceptability to patients, specialists and general practitioners', *Journal of Epidemiology and Community Health*, 51: 52–61.

Boyle, P.J., Kudlac, H. and Williams, A.J. (1996) 'Geographical variation in the referral of patients with chronic end stage renal failure for renal replacement therapy', *Quarterly Journal of Medicine*, 89: 151–7.

Brown, D.B. (1979) 'Proxy measures in accident countermeasure evaluation: a study of emergency medical services', *Journal of Safety Research*, 11: 37–41.

Campbell, N.C., Elliott, A.M., Sharp, L., Ritchie, L.D., Cassidy, J. and Little, J. (2000) 'Rural factors and survival from cancer: analysis of Scottish cancer registrations', *British Journal of Cancer*, 82: 1863–6.

Campbell, N.C., Ritchie, L.D., Cassidy, J. and Little, J. (1999) 'Systematic review of cancer treatment programmes in remote and rural areas', *British Journal of Cancer*, 80: 1275–80.

Carr-Hill, R.A., Place, M. and Posnett, J. (1997) 'Access and the utilisation of healthcare services'. In B. Ferguson, T. Sheldon and J. Posnett (eds) *Concentration and Choice in Healthcare*. London: Financial Times Healthcare.

Carr-Hill, R.A., Rice, N. and Roland, M. (1996) 'Socio-economic determinants of rates of consultation in general practice based on Fourth National Morbidity Survey of general practices', *British Medical Journal*, 312: 1008–1012.

Carr-Hill, R.A., Sheldon, T.A., Smith, P., Martin, S., Peacock, S. and Hardman, G. (1994) 'Allocating resources to health authorities: development of method for small area analysis of use of inpatient services', *British Medical Journal*, 309: 1046–9.

Cartwright, A. and Anderson, R. (1981) *General Practice Revisited*. London: Tavistock Publications.

Cloke, P., Goodwin, M., Milbourne, P. and Thomas, C. (1995) 'Deprivation, poverty and marginalization in rural lifestyles in England and Wales', *Journal of Rural Studies*, 11: 351–65.

Commission for Health Improvement (2001) *NHS Cancer Care in England and Wales*. London: Commission for Health Improvement.

Congdon, P. (2000) 'A Bayesian approach to prediction using the gravity model, with an application to patient care modelling', *Geographical Analysis*, 32: 205–24.

Countryside Agency (2001a) *Rural Services in 2000*. Cheltenham: Countryside Agency.

Countryside Agency (2001b) *The State of the Countryside 2001*. Cheltenham: Countryside Agency.

Cox, J. (1998) 'Poverty in rural areas', *British Medical Journal*, 316: 722.

Craft, P.S., Primrose, J.G., Lindner, J.A. and McManus P.R. (1997) 'Surgical management of breast cancer in Australian women in 1994', *Medical Journal of Australia*, 166: 626–9.

Cross, K.W. and Turner, R.D. (1974) 'Factors affecting the visiting pattern of geriatric patients in a rural area', *British Journal of Preventive and Social Medicine*, 28: 133–9.

Dalziel, M. and Garrett, C. (1987) 'Intraregional variation in treatment of end stage renal failure', *British Medical Journal*, 294: 1382–3.

Department for Environment, Food and Rural Affairs (2000) *Our Countryside: The Future. A Fair Deal for Rural England*. London: The Stationery Office.

Department of the Environment, Transport and the Regions (2000) *Transport 2010: The 10 Year Plan*. London: The Stationery Office.

Department of Health (1997) *The New NHS: Modern Dependable*, Cmnd 3807. London: HMSO.

Department of Health (1999a) *Reducing Health Inequalities: An Action Report*. London: Department of Health.

Department of Health (1999b) *Resource Allocation: Weighted Capitation Formulas*. London: Department of Health.

Department of Health (2000a) *The NHS Plan*, Cmnd 4818. London: The Stationery Office.

Department of Health (2000b) *The NHS Cancer Plan: A Plan for Investment, a Plan for Reform*. London: The Stationery Office.

Department of Health and Social Security (1976) *Sharing Resources for Health in England: Report of the Resource Allocation Working Party*. London: The Stationery Office.

Department of Health and Social Security (1980) *Report of the Working Group on Inequalities in Health* (Black Report). London: DHSS.

Dunn, N.R., Arscott, A., Thorogood, M., Faragher, B., de Caestecker, L. MacDonald, T.M., McCollum, C. Thomas, S. and Mann, R.D. (2000) 'Regional variation in incidence and case fatality of myocardial infarction among young women in England, Scotland and Wales', *Journal of Epidemiology and Community Health*, 54: 293–8.

Fearn, R. (1987) 'Rural health care: a British success or a tale of unmet need?', *Social Science and Medicine*, 24: 263–74.

Fearn, R.M.G., Haynes, R.M. and Bentham, C.G. (1984) 'Role of branch surgeries in a rural area', *Journal of the Royal College of General Practitioners*, 34: 488–91.

Feest, T.J., Mistry, C.D., Grimes, D.S., Mallick, N.P. (1990) 'Incidence of advanced chronic renal failure and the need for end stage renal replacement treatment', *British Medical Journal*, 301: 897–900.

Fylkesnes, K., Johnsoen, R. and Forde O.H. (1992) 'The Tromso study: factors affecting patient initiated and provider initiated use of health care services', *Sociology of Health and Illness*, 14: 275–92.

Garrett, J.E. (1997) 'Health service accessibility and deaths from asthma', *Thorax*, 52: 205–6.

Garrett, J., Mulder, J. and Wong-Toi, H. (1986) 'Characteristics of asthmatics using an urban accident and emergency department', *New Zealand Medical Journal*, 101: 359–61.

Gibson, D.M., Goodin, R.E. and LeGrand, J. (1985) 'Come and get it: distributional biases in social service delivery systems', *Policy and Politics*, 13: 109–25.

Gillam, S.J., Ball, M., Prasad, M., Dunne, H., Cohen, S. and Vafdis, G. (1995) 'Investigation of benefits and costs of an ophthalmic outreach clinic in general practice', *British Journal of General Practice*, 45: 649–52.

Goddard, M. and Smith, P. (1998) *Equity of access to health care*. York: Centre for Health Economics, University of York.

Greenberg, E.R., Chute, C.G., Stukel, T., Baron, J.A., Freeman, D.H., Yates, J. and Korson, R. (1988) 'Social and economic factors in the choice of lung cancer treatment', *New England Journal of Medicine*, 318: 612–7.

Haggett, P., Cliff, A.D. and Frey, A. (1977) *Locational Models*. London: Edward Arnold.

Haiart, D.C., McKenzie, L., Henderson, J., Pollock, W., McQueen, D.V., Roberts, M.M. and Forrest, A.P.M. (1990) 'Mobile breast screening: factors affecting uptake, efforts to increase response and acceptability', *Public Health*, 104: 239–47.

Hart, J.T. (1971) 'The inverse care law', *Lancet*, 1: 405–12.

Haynes, R.M. and Bentham, C.G. (1979) *Community Hospitals and Rural Accessibility*. Farnborough: Saxon House.

Haynes, R., Bentham, G., Lovett, A. and Gale, S. (1999) 'Effects of distances to hospital and GP surgery on hospital inpatient episodes, controlling for needs and provision', *Social Science and Medicine*, 49: 425–33.

Haynes, R. and Gale, S. (1999) 'Mortality, long term illness and deprivation in rural and metropolitan wards of England and Wales', *Health & Place*, 5: 301–12.

Haynes, R., Gale, S., Mugford, M. and Davies, D. (2001) 'Cataract surgery in a community hospital outreach clinic: patients' costs and satisfaction', *Social Science and Medicine*, 53: 1631–40.

Higgs, G. and White, S. (2000) 'Alternatives to census-based indicators of social disadvantage in rural communities', *Progress in Planning*, 53: 1–81.

Horrocks, S., Anderson, E. and Salisbury C. (2002) 'Systematic review of whether nurse practitioners working in primary care can provide equivalent care to doctors', *British Medical Journal*, 324: 819–23.

Jarman, B. (1983) 'Identification of under-privileged areas', *British Medical Journal*, 286: 1705–8.

Jarvis, E. (1850) 'The influence of distance from and proximity to an insane hospital, on its use by any people', *Boston Medical and Surgical Journal*, 42: 209–22.

Jones, A.P. and Bentham, G. (1995) 'Emergency medical service accessibility and outcome from road traffic accidents', *Public Health*, 109: 169–77.

Jones, A.P. and Bentham, G. (1997) 'Health service accessibility and deaths from asthma in 401 local authority districts in England and Wales, 1988–92', *Thorax*, 52: 218–22.

Jones, A.P., Bentham, G., Harrison, B.D.W., Jarvis, D., Badminton, R.M. and Wareham, N.J. (1998) 'Accessibility and health service utilization for asthma in Norfolk, England', *Journal of Public Health Medicine*, 20: 312–17.

Jones, A.P., Bentham, G. and Horwell, C. (1999) 'Health service accessibility and deaths from asthma', *International Journal of Epidemiology*, 28: 101–5.

Joseph A.E. and Bantock. P.R. (1982) 'Measuring potential physical accessibility to general practitioners in rural areas: a method and case study', *Social Science and Medicine*, 16: 85–90.

Joseph, A.E. and Phillips, D.R. (1984) *Accessibility and Utilization: Geographical Perspectives on Health Care Delivery*. London: Harper and Row.

Kim, Y.E., Gatrell, A.C. and Francis, B.J. (2000) 'The geography of survival after surgery for colorectal cancer in Southern England', *Social Science and Medicine*, 50: 1099–107.

Lattimer, V., George, S., Thompson, F., Thomas, E., Mullee, M., Turnbull, J., Smith, H., Moore, M., Bond, H. and Gasper, A. (1998) 'Safety and effectiveness of nurse telephone consultation in out of hours primary care; randomised controlled trial', *British Medical Journal*, 317: 1054–9.

Launoy, G., Le Coutour, X., Gignoux, M., Pottier, D. and Dugleux, G. (1992) 'Influence of rural environment on diagnosis, treatment and prognosis of colorectal cancer', *Journal of Epidemiology and Community Health*, 46: 365–7.

Liff, J.M., Chow, W.-H. and Greenberg, R.S. (1991) 'Rural–urban differences in stage at diagnosis: possible relationship to cancer screening', *Cancer*, 67: 1454–9.

London Health Planning Consortium Study Group (1981) *Primary Health Care in Inner London*. London: London Health Planning Consortium.

Longley, P.A., Goodchild, M.F., Maguire, D.J. and Rhind, D.W. (2001) *Geographic Information Systems and Science*. Chichester: Wiley.

Lovett, A., Haynes, R. and Sunnenberg, G. (1998) *Accessibility of Potential Sites for Intermediate Services*. Norwich: School of Environmental Sciences, University of East Anglia.

Lovett, A., Haynes, R., Sunnenberg, G. and Gale, S. (2000) *Accessibility of Primary Health Care Services in East Anglia*. Research Report 9, Norwich: School of Medicine, Health Policy and Practice, University of East Anglia.

Lovett, A., Haynes, R., Sunnenberg, G. and Gale, S. (2002) 'Car travel time and accessibility by bus to general practitioner services: a study using patient registers and GIS', *Social Science and Medicine*, 55: 97–111.

Martin, D. and Williams, H.C.W.L. (1992) 'Market area analysis and accessibility to primary health care centres', *Environment and Planning A*, 24: 1009–19.

Martin, D., Roderick, P., Diamond, I., Clements, S. and Stone, N. (1998) 'Geographical aspects of the uptake of renal replacement therapy in England', *International Journal of Population Geography*, 4: 227–42.

Martin, D., Senior, M.L. and Williams, H.C.W.L. (1994) 'On measures of deprivation and the spatial allocation of resources for primary health care', *Environment and Planning A*, 26: 1911–29.

Martin, D., Wrigley, H., Barnett, S. and Roderick, P. (2002) 'Increasing the sophistication of access measurement in a rural healthcare study', *Health and Place*, 8: 3–13.

McLaughlin, B. (1986) 'The rhetoric and reality of rural deprivation', *Journal of Rural Studies*, 2: 291–307.

Mead, N., Gosden, T. and Roland, M. (1998) 'Conclusions and key issues for the future'. In M. Roland and J. Shapiro (eds) *Specialist Outreach Clinics in General Practice*. Oxford: Radcliffe Medical Press.

Medical Practices Committee (2000) *Annual Report for 1999/2000*. London: Department of Health.

Ministry of Health (1962) *A Hospital Plan for England and Wales*, Cmnd 1604. London: HMSO.

Montella, M., Biondi, E., De Marco, M., Botti, G., Tatangelo, F., Capasso, I. and Marone, A. (1995) 'Sociodemographic factors associated with the diagnostic staging of breast cancer in southern Italy', *Cancer*, 76: 1585–90.

Moseley, M.J. (1979) *Accessibility: The Rural Challenge*. London: Methuen.

Murray, S.A., Graham, L.J.C. and Dlugolecka, M.J. (1995) 'How many general practitioners for 1433 patients?' *British Medical Journal*, 310: 100.

Nutley, S.D. (1980) 'Accessibility, mobility and transport-related welfare: the case of rural Wales', *Geoforum*, 11: 335–52.

Office of Population Censuses and Surveys (1990) *Mortality and Geography: a Review in the mid-1980s*. Series DS no. 9. London: HMSO.

Office of Population Censuses and Surveys (1995) *Morbidity Statistics from General Practice. Fourth National Study 1991–1992*. Series MB5 No. 3. London: HMSO.

Phibbs, C.S. and Luft, H.S. (1995) 'Correlation of travel time on roads versus straight line distance', *Medical Care Research and Review*, 52: 532–42.

Phillimore, P. and Reading, R. (1992) 'A rural advantage? Urban–rural health differences in Northern England', *Journal of Public Health Medicine*, 14: 290–9.

Reading, R., Langford, I.H., Haynes, R. and Lovett, A. (1999) 'Accidents to preschool children: comparing family and neighbourhood risk factors', *Social Science and Medicine*, 48: 321–30.

Roland, M. and Shapiro, J. (eds) (1998) *Specialist Outreach Clinics in General Practice*. Oxford: Radcliffe Medical Press.

Salisbury, C.J. (1989) 'How do people choose their doctor?', *British Medical Journal*, 299: 608–10.

Senior, M., Williams, H. and Higgs, G. (2000) 'Urban–rural mortality differentials: controlling for material deprivation', *Social Science and Medicine*, 51: 289–305.

Shucksmith, M., Roberts, D., Scott, D., Chapman, P. and Conway, E. (1996) *Disadvantage in Rural Areas*. London: Rural Development Commission.

Smith, P., Sheldon, T.A., Carr-Hill, R.A., Martin, S., Peacock, S. and Hardman, G. (1994) 'Allocating resources to health authorities: results and policy implications of small area analysis of use of inpatient services', *British Medical Journal*, 309: 1050–4.

Soper, J., and Jones, J.J. (1985) 'Cost effectiveness of surgery in small acute "local" hospitals', *Community Medicine*, 7: 257–64.

Sowden, A.J., Watt, I. and Sheldon, T.A. (1997) 'Volume of activity and healthcare quality: is there a link?'. In B. Ferguson, T. Sheldon and J. Posnett (eds) *Concentration and Choice in Healthcare*. London: Financial Times Healthcare.

Tacket, A.R. (1989) 'Equity and access: exploring the effects of hospital location on the population served – a case study in strategic planning', *Journal of the Operational Research Society*, 40: 1001–10.

Taytard, A., Tessier, J.F., Gervais, M., Gachie, J.P., Douet, C., Kombou, L., Vergeret, J. and Freour, P. (1990) 'Actual usage of medical facilities by asthmatics in two French settings: a preliminary study', *European Respiratory Journal*, 3: 856–60.

Tomlinson, B. (1992) *Report of the inquiry into London's health service, medical education and research*. London: HMSO.

Venning, P., Durie, A., Roland, M., Roberts, C. and Leese, B. (2000) 'Randomised controlled trial comparing cost effectiveness of general practitioners and nurse practitioners in primary care', *British Medical Journal*, 320: 1048–53.

Watt, I.S. (1995) 'Health needs of rural residents'. In J. Cox (ed) *Rural General Practice in the United Kingdom*, Occasional Paper 71. London: Royal College of General Practitioners.

Watt, I.S. and Sheldon, T.A. (1993) 'Rurality and resource allocation in the UK', *Health Policy*, 26: 19–27.

Whewell, J., Marsh, G.N. and McNay, R.A. (1983) 'Changing patterns of home visiting in the North of England', *British Medical Journal*, 286: 1259–61.

Will, E.J., Davenport, A. and Davison, A.M. (1987) 'Intraregional variation in treatment of end stage renal failure', *British Medical Journal*, 295: 443.

Woollett, S. (1990) *Counting the Rural Cost: The Case for a Rural Premium*. London: National Council for Voluntary Organisations.

Wootton, R. (1999) 'Telemedicine and isolated communities: a UK perspective', *Journal of Telemedicine and Telecare*, 5 supplement 2: 27–34.

Chapter 3

Equity and access to health care

Martin Gulliford

Introduction

Equity requires that access to health care is fairly and justly distributed. Achieving equity depends both on there being a generally accepted conception of a just distribution of health care, and on there being effective mechanisms to ensure that this is implemented in practice. This chapter does not attempt to discuss different conceptions of social justice; these have been summarised elsewhere (Gillon 1986; Rawls 1999; Bommier and Stecklov 2002). Instead, we assume that 'access to health care is every citizen's right and this ought not to be influenced by income and wealth' (Williams 1993: 291). This egalitarian approach has informed the development of publicly funded health systems in the United Kingdom and western Europe (van Doorslaer *et al.* 1993). In the UK, the National Health Service in its first fifty years of development was supported by a consensus that health care should be financed according to ability to pay but distributed according to need, thereby setting out equity objectives in terms of both financial contribution and access to care.

Braveman *et al.* (2001) described equity in health as 'an ethical value that may be operationally defined as striving to reduce systematic disparities in health between more and less advantaged social groups within and between countries' (p. 679). This description illustrates how the concept of equity incorporates elements of both fact and value. Inequities are inequalities that are considered to be unjust or unfair (Pan American Health Organisation 2001). As there are sizeable inequalities in health and the need for health care in most societies, equality of access to health care will be unfair. According to the approach outlined above, social justice will be achieved if health care is distributed according to need (Gillon 1986).

An egalitarian approach is not universally accepted. The existence of a private sector in health care allows those who are able or willing to pay, to purchase additional access to health care. Here, notions of individual autonomy or freedom of choice seem to take precedence over equity of access. Existing health systems are pluralistic in the sense that they seem to accommodate differing ideologies with conflicting objectives (Williams 1993). Amy Gutmann (1981) observed that it is not surprising that equitable access to health care is not realised, when most institutions and services in society are far from egalitarian. If substantial inequalities in education, income and wealth are acceptable, equity in access to health care is unlikely to be attainable.

If equity is an ideal, then it is possible to measure the extent of departures from this and to use these to inform the development of policies. This chapter is therefore concerned with methods for describing and analysing the distribution of access to health care in populations. It is mainly concerned with the distribution of access according to characteristics such as health needs, socio-economic measures or ethnicity. The geographical or spatial distribution of access is discussed in Chapter 2, the position of marginalised and socially excluded groups is discussed in Chapter 4, and the role of private health care is discussed in Chapter 6.

The chapter begins by reviewing the meaning and measurement of equity in access to health care. It goes on to discuss two main groups of studies. The first has been implemented mainly by economists and has played an important role in clarifying the definition and measurement of equity (van Doorslaer *et al.* 1993). These studies have mostly used generic measures of health care need and utilisation, and will be referred to as 'generic' studies. The second group of studies has been implemented by a broader range of health services researchers, and aims to document inequalities and inequities in access to health care for specific conditions or services using condition-specific measures. These will be referred to as 'specific' studies. The findings from the two areas of work will be contrasted.

Definition and measurement of equity in access to health care

Equity in health care funding and access: horizontal and vertical dimensions

In the context of health care, the term equity may be applied either to health care access or to funding. Equity in the funding of health care exists when contributions are made according to ability to pay, while equity in access to health care exists when health care is accessed according to need. Both types of equity have a horizontal and a vertical dimension. Horizontal equity requires that equals are treated equally, while vertical equity requires that unequals are treated in proportion to their inequality (Gillon 1986). Vertical equity has received more attention in the funding of health care. Here, a central aim is to ensure that those with differing ability to pay, contribute in proportion to their differing income or wealth. Equity in the funding of health care has been discussed by Wagstaff *et al.* (1999) and this has direct implications for access (see Chapter 6). Horizontal equity has received more attention in access to health care, where ensuring that those with equal needs are treated equally is a key aim. In reality, different population groups usually have differing rather than equal needs. Mooney (2000) has suggested that addressing vertical equity in the delivery of health care, ensuring that groups with different needs receive appropriately differentiated treatment, may be a more important route to addressing existing inequalities in health.

Horizontal equity in access to health care

Horizontal equity in access to care requires that there is equal access to health care for those with equivalent needs. This principle may be applied to each of the three proposed measures of access: service availability, service utilisation or health outcomes. The concept of service availability may be extended here to include the distribution of all health care resources. Culyer and Wagstaff (1993) argued that equity in health outcomes is the most important measure of equity because this reflects the objective of health care provision, which is to improve health. In terms of heath policy, however, there seems to be a moderately strong consensus that public health care resources should be distributed equitably, so providing equivalent opportunities to access health care, but the commitment to equity in health itself appears to be relatively weak.

According to most definitions, equity is concerned with the relationship between health care needs and access to health care for different groups in the population. A widely accepted definition of need is capacity to benefit from health care (for example, Stevens and Raftery 1994). This definition encompasses not just the existence of a health problem but the possibility of intervening so as to improve health. Culyer and Wagstaff (1993) refined this definition to describe need as the expenditure required to effect the maximal possible health improvement. However, in practical terms needs are more often measured in terms of health status. Most generic evaluations of equity have used self-reported measures of health status. These typically include questions concerning self-rated health, or the presence or absence of self-reported short- or long-term illness, with or without limitation of activities (van Doorslaer et al. 2000). Condition-specific studies have employed combinations of generic and condition-specific health measurement scales (Gulliford and Mahabir 2001) or measures of clinical morbidity (Dong et al. 1998). These have the advantage of greater precision, but may not allow comparison between groups with different conditions.

The use of health status as an indicator of need for health care depends on the assumption that health status and need are consistently associated. Thus it is assumed that two groups with the same health status will have the same needs for services, or if the rate of ill-health is twice as high in one group as compared with another then the need for health care will be twice as great. These assumptions will not always be justified. There is also a difficulty in using subjective health measures as indicators of need because it is usually argued that needs should be assessed objectively. Subjective assessments represent patients' 'wants' rather than needs. The use of self-assessed health presents particular problems because it is not directly linked to an objective of health care delivery. Systematic differences in reporting by different groups also presents problems. An example given by Mooney et al. (2002) illustrates the type of problem that may arise. Aboriginal

Australians have a life expectancy that is fifteen to twenty years less than for Australians in general but, in a sample survey, 88 per cent of the Aboriginal group rated their health as being 'good', 'very good' or 'excellent' compared with 79 per cent of the general population. Within cultures there is known to be differential reporting of health status; for example, older people generally rate their health more favourably than younger people.

Evaluations of equity often ignore a distinction between the initial state of health, and the final state of health after receiving health care (Culyer 1993). Cross-sectional data do not allow health needs and health outcomes to be distinguished and will often be less suitable than longitudinal designs for the assessment of equity. This distinction is important if assessment of health outcomes is considered relevant to the evaluation of equity. Probably the majority of evaluations of equity have been based on cross-sectional data. Here it is not possible to relate health service utilisation to the state of health prior to contact with health services. This may lead to bias particularly when self-reported health measures are used (Sutton *et al.* 1999) because attendance at a medical consultation may alter subjects' reporting of illness. In chronic conditions, even longitudinal data may be difficult to interpret when health care may be accessed over a long period of time.

Social inequalities in health

Socio-economic status is associated with gradations in health status, and needs for health care. Evidence from many sources shows that at all ages people with lower socio-economic status are more likely to die, to suffer from specific diseases, or to experience illness or disability. These gradations may be observed with some variations, when people or populations are ranked according to income, employ-ment status, occupational social class, educational attainment or household amenities (Drever and Whitehead 1997; Davey Smith 1997). For example, in men aged 20 to 64 years in England and Wales all-cause mortality for those in unskilled occupations is 2.9 times higher than for those in professional occupations. Mortality from lung cancer is 4.8 times higher, mortality from accidents, poisoning and violence is 4.0 times higher and mortality from suicide and undetermined injury is 3.6 times higher (Acheson 1998). These social inequalities in health exist in most countries although there are variations in the size of inequalities for specific diseases (Kunst *et al.* 1998). Lower socio-economic status is associated with a greater need for health care and a lower ability to pay. In addition, knowledge of services, access to information and communication resources, or transport mobility, all of which facilitate access to health care, may be lower for groups with lower socio-economic status. In evaluating equity, it is essential that socio-economic inequalities in access to care are judged in relation to socio-economic inequalities in health.

Ethnic minority groups in Europe, the USA and Australasia experience socio-economic disadvantage. There are also distinct ethnic variations in the distribution of specific health conditions. A minority of these conditions, such as sickle cell disease, have well defined genetic causes. More often, as in the case of diabetes or psychoses, the causes are more complex and may include material deprivation, cultural factors, selection through migration, the consequences of migration and discrimination, as well as possible genetic factors (Smaje 1995). Inequalities in health between ethnic groups cannot be ascribed only to socio-economic factors or to supposed 'ethnic factors'; rather, there are complex inter-relationships between ethnicity and socio-economic status which may vary for different health outcomes (Davey Smith 2000). In relation to access, differences in language or culture, and real or perceived discrimination by providers, may present barriers to health care. A growing body of work has therefore attempted to evaluate horizontal equity in relation to ethnicity. Here it is necessary to adjust measures of access for health needs, and relevant socio-economic characteristics, in order to determine whether there are inequities in relation to ethnicity.

Many studies of socio-economic or ethnic inequalities in health or health care utilisation have relied on individual-level data to describe social characteristics. The availability of census-derived and other data to describe the socio-economic characteristics of small areas, together with the development of methods of analysis for multilevel data structures, has led to increasing interest in possible area-level effects on health. Does the 'context' in terms of the local physical or social environment have an influence on health after allowing for the 'composition' of the population measured according to individual characteristics? Some studies suggest that there are significant area-level contextual effects, but little work has been done to understand why such contextual effects exist, or to test different potential explanations (Macintyre *et al.* 2002). Area effects are particularly relevant to the assessment of inequity because geographical inequalities in service availability are themselves associated with socio-economic status. However, few studies to date have used a multilevel approach to the evaluation of equity.

Assessment of inequality and inequity

Inequalities in health provide the context in which equity in access to health care must be judged. Particular attention has been given to developing appropriate methods of estimating inequalities in health and differentials in access among social groups. Reviews are provided by Wagstaff *et al.* (1991), Mackenbach and Kunst (1997), and Manor *et al.* (1997). There are three basic approaches that depend on simple comparison of rates of access for different groups, on the use of regression methods, or on the development of Gini-like coefficients. Details of calculations are provided by Mackenbach and Kunst (1997).

Comparison of rates

Rates of access may be compared for different population groups. Either an absolute measure, the difference in rates between the selected group and the reference group, or a relative measure, the ratio of rates between selected and reference groups, may be used for presentation. In terms of socio-economic status, the groups of interest may be defined according to percentiles of the distribution (of income say) or in terms of a standard classification such as the Registrar General's classification of social class. In order to estimate the total impact of socio-economic inequalities on a population's access to health care, it is necessary to take into account the relative size of different socio-economic groups. This can be done by estimating the population-attributable risk, which provides an estimate of the overall increase in access that would be achieved if the whole population enjoyed the same level of access as that obtained by those in the highest socio-economic category (Mackenbach and Kunst 1997).

Early approaches to the evaluation of equity relied on these simple quantitative comparisons of need and health care utilisation in different socio-economic groups, in the form of 'use–needs ratios'. Le Grand (1978) used data from the General Household Survey in England and Wales to see if the proportion of health care utilisation by different socio-economic groups was in proportion to their share of self-reported illness. This approach was extended by Collins and Klein (1980) who separated different needs groups, as well as socio-economic groups. These groups included those reporting no ill health, those reporting acute sickness, and those reporting long-term sickness with or without limitations on their activities. This distinction was considered important because different social groups might vary in their pattern of health care utilisation in relation to need. In particular, it was not justified to assume that people who did not report illness did not utilise health care.

Regression methods

Regression methods offer an alternative method for contrasting groups of interest through the estimation of regression coefficients and odds ratios. Regression methods may be used to produce overall summary measures of inequality in access. This usually requires an assumption that the chosen measure of socio-economic status represents an interval scale. For example, a regression model can be used to estimate the change in access for each additional year spent in full-time education, or for each £1,000 increase in household income. The slope index of inequality can be estimated using a similar approach. Here, the cumulative proportion of the population in each socio-economic category is estimated, and the mid-point for each category is fitted as predictor that theoretically ranges from 0 to 1. The regression coefficient (the slope index of inequality) then represents the difference in access between those at the top and those at the bottom of the socio-economic scale (Mackenbach and Kunst 1997).

Regression methods can be used to evaluate inequity in access to health care by permitting analysis of individual-level data for access, according to socio-economic group, after standardising for need. The dependent variable is the chosen measure of access which may reflect service availability, utilisation or outcome.

Explanatory variables include measures of health need (for example, in need or not) and socio-economic status (for example, income, education or employment) for each individual. Relevant demographic variables such as age and sex may also be included as explanatory variables. The regression coefficient for socio-economic status provides a measure of the mean difference in access between social groups after adjusting for need. Appropriate interaction terms may also be evaluated to allow for the possibility that the relationship between need and access varies in different socio-economic groups. In this model if, after adjusting for needs and demographic variables, access is explained by socio-economic status, there is evidence of inequity (Wagstaff *et al.* 1991). The regression coefficient can be used to test and quantify the degree of inequity between socio-economic groups.

Gini-like coefficients

Indices adapted from the Gini coefficient are being increasingly applied to health data. The Gini coefficient is derived from the Lorenz curve which describes the distribution of income in a population. The Gini coefficient provides a measure of income inequality. Similarly, a Gini coefficient can be estimated to summarise inequality in the distribution of health (or health care access) in a population. An index adapted from the Gini coefficient was included in the World Health Report 2000 (World Health Organisation 2000) to describe health inequalities in different countries. This has been criticised because it failed to take into account the socio-economic dimension of health inequalities (for example Braveman *et al.* 2001; Szwarcwald 2002). As Wagstaff *et al.* (1991) have pointed out, the Gini index as a measure of health inequality will show a decrease even when any reduction in ill health is confined to the more affluent. This is because the index does not include the dimension of socio-economic status. Murray *et al.* (2001) have argued that health inequalities are of interest whatever their cause, but others (for example Wagstaff *et al.* 1991a; Braveman *et al.* 2001) suggest that what is concerning about health inequalities is that they parallel socio-economic inequalities in most societies.

Van Doorslaer *et al.* (1993, 2000) estimated measures of inequity based on the concentration index. The concentration index is adapted from the Gini index approach. In this application, the cumulative proportion of the population, ranked by income, is plotted on the horizontal axis. The cumulative proportion of either health care utilisation or need is plotted on the vertical axis. The concentration curve therefore describes the distribution of income-related inequalities in need or access. The diagonal line represents a situation of equal distribution of health care utilisation or need (Figure 3.1). When the poor have a lower share of health care utilisation (or need) than the rich, the curve will lie below the diagonal but when there is inequality giving a greater share of need or utilisation to the poor, the curve will lie above the diagonal. The concentration index is estimated as twice the area between the concentration curve and the diagonal. It will have a value of 0 when there is no inequality, and a value of 1 where there is maximum

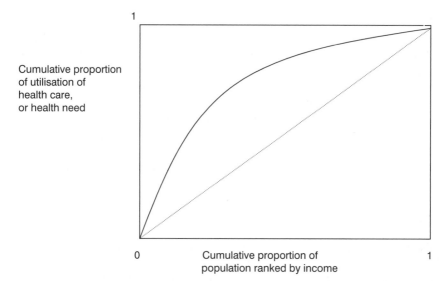

Figure 3.1 Showing inequality in the distribution of utilisation of health care, or need, favouring the poor

inequality. A positive value indicates inequality favouring the rich, and a negative value indicates inequality favouring the poor. The distribution of need will usually be concentrated towards the poor. Horizontal equity requires that the distribution of health care utilisation is consistent with the distribution of need.

In order to evaluate horizontal inequity, the expected level of health care utilisation for each income group, based on its share of need, can be estimated by indirect standardisation using the distribution of utilisation by need in the whole sample for reference. The concentration curve for observed utilisation can be compared with a second concentration curve for expected utilisation after standardising for need. The index of horizontal inequity proposed by van Doorslaer *et al.* (2000) is given by the difference between the concentration indices for observed utilisation and expected utilisation after standardising for need. A positive value is consistent with horizontal inequity in the utilisation of health care favouring the more affluent, and a negative value indicates inequity favouring the poor.

The concentration index approach is being applied increasingly in the assessment of inequalities and inequities in health care access. For example, Lorant *et al.* (2002) analysed data from a health interview survey in Belgium. Subjects were ranked according to an index of socio-economic status that was based on income, education, occupation and housing tenure. Concentration indices were estimated for need (based on age, sex, self-rated health measures and self-reported illnesses) and for utilisation of health care (including primary, secondary and preventive health care).

Choice of measure

Which measures of inequality in access should be preferred? Mackenbach and Kunst (1997) suggest that it may be necessary to present results obtained using several methods. These should include both absolute and relative measures of access, and estimates obtained through simple comparisons of rates and from more sophisticated methods based on regression or the estimation of Gini-like coefficients. Simpler methods are often easier to interpret but make less efficient use of the data available. Regression methods and Gini-like coefficients make better use of the data, but provide measures which are less easy to interpret. The limitations of the assumptions underlying application of these methods may also be less obvious.

Summary

Horizontal inequities in access to health care may be estimated by using appropriate measures to quantify access, need, and socio-economic status (or other measures of inequality). Differences between groups in needs-standardised measures of access quantify the degree of horizontal inequity between groups. Measures of need and access for different groups in the population may also be plotted in the form of concentration curves, and a concentration index may be used to summarise the overall extent of inequity.

Evidence of inequity

The following sections discuss evidence of inequity in access to health care. The discussion is limited to inequity in relation to socio-economic status and ethnicity; other dimensions for evaluation were reviewed by Goddard and Smith (2001). In addition to systematic inequities in access to services, there are well documented but seemingly random variations in the availability and use of services which must often be considered inequitable. The results of generic studies are described first, and then contrasted with the results of studies in specific conditions and client groups. While generic studies address equity at the level of the health care system, specific studies are more concerned with evaluating equity in clinical services.

Assessment of horizontal inequity in generic studies

Several generic evaluations of horizontal equity in access to health care have been reported (see Table 3.1). These evaluations were based on data from general purpose or health interview surveys. Access to health care was generally measured in terms of self-reported utilisation of health care during a defined period of time; health needs were assessed using data for self-assessed health or self-reported acute or long-term sickness, with or without limitation of activities; socio-economic status was measured in terms of occupational social class or self-reported

Table 3.1 Findings of generic evaluations of horizontal inequity in utilisation of health care in the UK

Author (year)	Data	Methods	Health services	Main findings
Socio-economic status				
Le Grand (1978)	GHS	Use/needs ratios	Overall	Pro-rich inequity
Collins and Klein (1980)	GHS	Use/needs ratios	Primary care	No inequity overall
Puffer (1986)	GHS	Regression	Primary care	No inequity overall, some evidence for pro-rich inequity in women only
O'Donnell and Propper (1991)	GHS	Regression	No inequity overall	
Van Doorslaer et al. (1993)	GHS	Regression	Primary care Inpatient, Outpatient	No inequity
Smaje and Le Grand (1997)	GHS	Use/needs ratios Regression	Primary care Inpatient, Outpatient	Pro-poor inequity
Whitehead et al. (1997)	GHS	Regression	Primary care, Outpatient	Pro-poor inequity in primary care use, not in use of hospital services
Cooper et al. (1998)	GHS children	Regression	Primary care Inpatient, Outpatient	No inequity
Cooper et al. (1999)	GHS children	Regression	Primary care Inpatient, Outpatient	No inequity
Van Doorslaer et al. (2000)	GHS	Concentration index	Primary care Inpatient, Outpatient	No inequity overall, some pro-rich inequity in use of specialist care
Ethnicity				
Smaje and Le Grand (1997)	GHS	Use/needs ratios Regression	Primary care Inpatient, Outpatient	Pro-minority in primary care, pro-majority in use of hospital services
Cooper et al. (1998)	GHS children	Regression	Primary care Inpatient, Outpatient	Pro-minority in primary care, pro-majority in use of hospital services
Cooper et al. (1999)	GHS children	Regression	Primary care Inpatient, Outpatient	Pro-minority in primary care, pro-majority in use of hospital services

household income. The studies differed in the methods used to combine these variables.

Socio-economic status

Le Grand (1978) used data from the General Household Survey in England and Wales to estimate the proportion of each social class group reporting either limiting longstanding illness or acute sickness. After standardising for age and sex, 15 per cent of social class I and II (professional and managerial) reported these indicators of need compared with 29 per cent of social class IV and V (semi-skilled and unskilled manual). The distribution of health care expenditure was calculated from reported utilisation of GP consultations, hospital outpatient visits, and hospital inpatient days. The proportion of health care expenditure ranged from 19 per cent in social class I and II to 26 per cent in social class IV and V. The ratio of expenditure per person reporting ill in social class I and II, compared with social class IV and V, was 1.4. This result indicated inequity favouring the more affluent. The methods used by Le Grand were criticised because his approach assumed that the non-sick did not need or utilise health care. This would lead to a bias in favour of the rich, because this group has the largest proportion of non-sick.

Collins and Klein (1980) used tabulation methods to analyse the General Household Survey data. They found that in people who did not report illness, rates of contacts with primary care doctors were similar in professional (men 7.0 per cent, women 7.5 per cent) and unskilled manual groups (men 5.4 per cent, women 8.5 per cent) with no obvious gradient according to social class. In those reporting acute illness, primary care use by men in unskilled manual groups (71.0 per cent) tended to be higher than for professionals (40.9 per cent) but this was not so for women. The authors suggested that this finding might be explained by the need to obtain sickness absence certificates. In subjects reporting chronic illness without restrictions, there was also a trend to greater utilisation of primary care by men in lower socio-economic groups (professional 7.1 per cent, unskilled manual 14.6 per cent). The results seemed to exclude inequity favouring the more affluent in the utilisation of primary care.

Van Doorslaer et al. (1993) used the concentration index approach to evaluate inequity in the utilisation of health care in the UK and other European countries. In a recent report, van Doorslaer et al. (2000) described analyses of data from household surveys in eleven countries. Inequities were evaluated in relation to household income. In all countries, the distribution of the utilisation of health care was weighted towards lower-income groups (values for the concentration index were negative in all countries and for different types of care). However, after standardising for age, sex and the indicators of need, values for the index of horizontal inequity were less negative. Simultaneous adjustment for self-assessed health and chronic illness gave values which were less negative than those obtained with either variable separately. This result suggested that after more complete adjustment for need, there was reduced evidence of inequity favouring the poor.

After adjustment for all needs variables there was evidence of pro-rich inequity in the distribution of doctor visits for five of the countries (US, Sweden, Finland, Netherlands and East Germany) but not in five other countries (Belgium, Denmark, West Germany, Switzerland or UK). Pro-rich inequity appeared to result from greater utilisation of specialist rather than primary care physician contacts among the more affluent. There was no significant inequity with respect to hospital in-patient days (except for pro-poor bias in the UK) or with respect to aggregated health care expenditure. The authors concluded that despite a pro-poor bias in the utilisation of most forms of medical care, after adjusting for need there was 'little evidence of an inequitable overall health care distribution' although there was some evidence of a pro-rich bias in the utilisation of specialist care in some countries (van Doorslaer et al. 2000: 581).

More recent analyses from the same group have been based on the European Community Household Panel which provides data collected using standard methods for twelve European Union member states. These results show that there was mostly equitable utilisation of general practitioner visits, but there was significant pro-rich inequity in the utilisation of visits to specialists in all of the countries except Luxembourg which only provided a small sample (van Doorslaer et al. 2002). The findings draw attention to possible systematic differences in the setting in which care is received by different groups. A partial explanation for the increased use of specialist care by more affluent groups is that they may be able to supplement access to the public system by purchasing private health insurance. This 'double coverage' may enhance access to specialist care (van Doorslaer et al. 2002). These observations show that even when there is an apparently equitable overall distribution of health care, there may be differential utilisation of types care which may differ in terms of quality.

Ethnicity

Generic studies using data from the British General Household Survey have given fairly consistent results across age groups (see Table 3.1). In general, ethnic minority groups are higher users of primary care services but show lower utilisation of hospital outpatient or inpatient services than white Europeans. For example, Smaje and Le Grand (1997) compared utilisation of services by ethnic minority groups with those of 'white' European subjects. In those under 45 years, odds ratios for use of primary care, after adjusting for age, sex and 'need', were 1.17 for 'Pakistanis' and 1.18 for 'Caribbean' people, indicating relatively higher rates of utilisation. These estimates were judged to be statistically 'significant' and not explained by additional adjustment for socio-economic status. There were interactions with gender such that 'Pakistani' women were less frequent consulters, while 'Caribbean' women were more frequent consulters than 'white' women. However, equivalent odds ratios for use of outpatient consultations were 0.59 for 'Pakistanis', 0.61 for 'Indians' and 0.63 for 'Caribbeans', indicating relatively lower rates of utilisation. These findings are broadly consistent across all ethnic minority groups studied, although people classified as 'Chinese' showed reduced overall health care utilisation in relation to need. These findings are difficult to interpret, but suggest some inequity in utilisation of hospital services, while there is more than equitable utilisation of primary care services. One explanation may be that ethnic minorities have access to lower-quality primary care services, leading to a higher consultation rate (Goddard and Smith 2001).

Limitations of generic studies

The findings from generic studies in horizontal equity are perhaps surprising because the structural characteristics of health care systems in some countries, notably the USA, are considered to be highly inequitable (Reinhardt 1996). It is relevant to consider the limitations of these studies. First, misclassification errors in the assessment of health care needs and health care utilisation may give a bias against the detection of inequity. O'Donnell and Propper (1991) discussed evidence from the Health and Lifestyle Survey which showed that among people reporting limiting longstanding illness, those from lower socio-economic groups were more likely to have more than one condition, and they reported more serious or severe conditions than those in higher socio-economic groups. Sutton *et al.* (1999) also found that errors in self-reported health measures could lead to substantial under-estimation of differences in health status between groups. In the assessment of horizontal equity, this would result in a bias against the detection of inequity, favouring the rich, because the health needs of poorer groups would be under-estimated. Second, these studies only evaluated utilisation of services and did not consider service availability and outcomes. Self-reported utilisation measures only summarise contacts with services and do not describe the technical content of care, including the outcomes achieved. It may be unlikely that the care received by the poor is equivalent in quality to that received by the rich, especially because health outcomes are worse among the poor. Third, measures of income or socio-economic status must be viewed in the context of the services available (see Chapter 2). For example, in rural areas car-ownership may be important in facilitating access to health care (Haynes 1991). Evaluation of possible contextual effects require modelling at more than one level. Fourth, generic studies generally assume that differentials of socio-economic status or income divide an otherwise homogenous population. Vulnerable groups with special needs deserve to be considered separately. More detailed studies of specific conditions and their treatment are needed in order to address these issues.

Assessment of horizontal equity in specific studies: documentation of the 'inverse care law'

In 1971, Julian Tudor Hart described what he termed the 'inverse care law'. He argued that 'the availability of good medical care tends to vary inversely with the need for it in the population served' (Tudor Hart 1971: 405). He went on in areas with the most sickness and death, general practitioners have more work, larger lists, less hospital support, and inherit more clinically ineffective traditions of consultation, than in the healthiest areas; and hospital doctors shoulder heavier case-loads with less staff and equipment, more obsolete buildings and suffer recurrent crises in the availability of beds and replacement staff.

(Tudor Hart 1971: 405)

Tudor Hart's analysis suggested that there were widespread inequities in access to both primary and secondary health care. Over the last three decades many specific studies both in Britain and in other countries have claimed to provide empirical evidence for the 'inverse care law'. Writing in 2001, Tudor Hart (2001) claimed: 'the inverse care law literature ... has created a mountain of supportive empirical evidence, which my original paper largely lacked' (pp. 18–19).

Primary care

There are well documented inequalities in the availability of general practitioners in England. Gravelle and Sutton (2001) found that the number of GPs per 10,000 population in administrative areas in England ranged from approximately 3.5 to 8.0 in 1995. Analysis of data for the ninety-nine health authorities in England for 1999 (Department of Health 2001a) shows a strong negative correlation between the Townsend deprivation score and the number of whole time equivalent general practitioners per 10,000 population. More deprived areas with higher Townsend scores have fewer general practitioners. Areas with fewer doctors are generally inner city areas with deprived populations generating a high workload but with few amenities to attract doctors. These inequalities have persisted, with some reduction, in spite of the introduction of policies designed to correct them (see Chapter 2). Similar variations have been documented in other countries including Spain (Abasolo et al. 2001) and the USA (Shi and Starfield 2001). As well as having fewer doctors, the structural characteristics of practices in deprived areas differ from those in more affluent areas. Practices in deprived areas are more likely to be 'single-handed' or to have older doctors, have less well developed facilities and provide fewer services (Leese and Bosanquet 1995). For example, practices in deprived areas are less likely to organise health promotion clinics (Gillam 1992); they are less likely to have on-site access to dietitian or chiropodist advice for diabetic patients (Khunti et al. 2001); they offer shorter consultation times (Stirling et al. 2001); and they obtain fewer funds for staff education and training (Hull et al. 2000).

Utilisation of primary care services is high in deprived areas. Salisbury et al. (2000) found that patients living in deprived areas made 70 per cent more calls to out-of-hours primary care services than those in non-deprived areas. In addition, deprived areas show increased utilisation of hospital accident and emergency services (Carlisle et al. 2000). These findings could be partly explained by higher levels of health need and by different patterns of help-seeking behaviour (see Chapter 4), but there is also evidence to suggest that the quality of primary care services is less satisfactory in deprived areas. For example, patients attending practices in deprived areas tend to be less satisfied with their care overall, and with interpersonal aspects of care in particular (Campbell *et al.* 2001). Children living in deprived areas are less likely to have their respiratory symptoms diagnosed as asthma, and are less likely to receive appropriate medication (Duran-Tauleria *et al.* 1996). If such examples are generalised they might contribute to higher consultation rates.

Some of the largest inequalities and inequities may relate to the utilisation of preventive medical care. In the UK, practices with more deprived populations show lower uptake of cervical screening (Majeed *et al.* 1994) and childhood immunisation (Lynch 1995). In a study from Belgium, Lorant *et al.* (2002) found that there was substantial pro-poor inequity in the utilisation of general practitioner services, but striking pro-rich inequity in the utilisation of preventive medical care including flu vaccination, cholesterol screening, mammography, and cervical smears. The authors observed that because uptake of preventive medicine is more inequitable than overall utilisation of health care, promoting screening has the potential to increase health inequalities.

It is well known that deprived areas show worse health than more affluent areas. Shi and Starfield (2001) recently suggested that lack of access to adequate primary health care in more deprived areas may be contributing to worse population health outcomes in the USA. In an ecological analysis of data for fifty US states, they found that after adjusting for income inequality and smoking, the total age-adjusted mortality rate decreased by 22.9 (95 per cent confidence interval 4.5 to 41.3) per 100,000 for each unit increase in the number of primary care physicians per 10,000 population (Shi *et al.* 1999). They suggested that effective primary care services may have some effect at mitigating the effect of poverty on health. Equivalent analyses for data for English health authorities showed a similar relationship between higher primary care physician supply and lower mortality but this was not entirely independent of adjustment for area-based measures of socio-economic status (Gulliford 2002).

Current thinking gives greater importance to the wider determinants of population health, but Bunker *et al.* (1994) suggested that medical care may contribute to as much as five years of present life expectancy. Bunker *et al.* pointed out that there was potential for a further gain in life expectancy if effective treatments were implemented more comprehensively. One recent systematic review found that there were serious problems with the quality of primary health care. Even the best performing practices sometimes only conform to recommended standards of care on less than 50 per cent of occasions (Seddon *et al.* 2001). Thus it is possible that inequalities in access to good-quality primary care may have some influence on population health. This has led to a growing interest in evaluating interventions to improve access to primary care services for disadvantaged groups (see Paterson and Judge, 2002 for review).

Hospital care

There is a widely accepted view that, at its outset, the NHS inherited a highly inequitable distribution of hospital services. Powell (1992) argued that this was only true for the voluntary hospital sector. When municipal hospital provision was included so as to estimate total hospital provision, Powell found there was little inequity in the distribution of hospital beds, but there was some inequity in the distribution of staff. The work of the Resource Allocation Working Party and its successors has attempted to move the pattern of allocation of resources to different areas, from one driven by historical patterns of supply, towards one more aligned with population size weighted for need (Smith *et al.* 1994) (see Chapter 2). Judge and Mays (1994) commented that the exclusion of resources for social care and primary health care from the resource allocation formula may contribute to inequity because areas with fewer primary care resources make higher demands on hospital services which are not accounted for in the formula. There is also a lack of transparency in the allocation of resources to different services and client groups at the local level. For example, many health authorities fail to achieve expected allocations for mental health services (Bindman *et al.* 2000). Current policies attempt to address these problems by including primary care resources within resource allocation formulae (Department of Health 2000) and devolving the commissioning role to primary care trusts (Department of Health 2001b).

Deprived areas show increased utilisation of hospital inpatient services but some studies suggest that there is inequity in the utilisation of specialist care. However, in contrast to the situation in the US where a consistent body of evidence shows that deprived and minority groups have lower access to specialist medical care, evidence from the UK is less consistent overall (Acheson 1998) (see Chapter 7). Access to specialist cardiac services represents one of the best investigated services. Here there is evidence that people living in more deprived areas are more likely to have symptomatic coronary artery disease but are less likely to receive investigation or treatment. Payne and Saul (1997) found that in more affluent electoral wards in Sheffield, 11 per cent of subjects with angina symptoms had coronary angiograms compared with 4 per cent in poorer electoral wards. Hippisley-Cox and Pringle (2000) studied general practices in the Trent region and found that the relative rate for coronary artery bypass surgery and angioplasty decreased by 1.2 per cent (95 per cent confidence interval 0.9 per cent to 1.5 per cent) for each unit increase in the Jarman under-privileged area score. When patients in more deprived areas are referred for surgery, they are less likely to be classed as 'urgent' cases and wait three weeks longer on average before receiving their operation (Pell *et al.* 2000). In the UK, people of Indian sub-continent origin who develop chest pain seem to experience longer delays and are less likely to receive thrombolytic treatment (Chaturvedi *et al.* 1997). Feder *et al.* (2002) found that among patients who were judged to need coronary revascularisation, people of Indian sub-continent descent were less likely to receive operations (age-adjusted hazard ratio compared with 'whites' 0.74, 95 per cent confidence interval 0.58 to

0.91). This difference was explained by adjusting for education and income either singly or in combination.

In a review of studies of gender bias in the utilisation of coronary artery disease treatment services, Raine (2000) highlighted some of the methodological limitations of specific studies of inequity in health care utilisation. Among thirteen studies which compared the use of coronary artery bypass surgery in men and women, four studied small samples (less than 1,000 subjects), three failed to explicitly define the condition being studied, none of the studies defined other risk factors such as comorbidity, and seven studies failed to use any form of adjustment for risk or need (Raine 2000). Goddard and Smith (2001) confirmed that many specific studies failed to adjust for need and therefore failed to distinguish between inequality and inequity. A further difficulty is that many UK studies have only included utilisation data from the NHS without including activity in the private sector (see Chapter 6). In view of these limitations, it is perhaps not surprising that the overall evidence is inconsistent and inconclusive (Goddard and Smith 2001). Selective publication and citation of this type of evidence may present a further problem. Systematic reviews are needed across a range of different areas of health care in order to evaluate the strength and consistency of the evidence of inequity in access to health care.

Do socio-economic differentials in access to hospital care lead on to differences in health outcomes? This question has been investigated in relation to several medical conditions. Data from the WHO MONICA study have been analysed to explore socio-economic inequalities in the case fatality of patients with myocardial infarction. Data from the Glasgow centre were analysed according to the Carstairs score for postcode sector of residence (Morrison *et al.* 1997). The incidence of myocardial infarction was 1.7 times higher in men, and 2.4 times higher in women, in the most deprived quartile compared with the least deprived quartile. However, the proportion of patients treated in hospital was lowest (age-standardised odds ratio 0.82) for the most deprived quartile. For hospitalised patients there was no overall socio-economic gradient in case fatality, but in the population as a whole the case fatality was highest in the most deprived quartile (age-standardised odds ratio 1.12 in men and 1.18 in women). Generally similar findings have been reported from other MONICA centres (Lang *et al.* 1998). Thus although incidence and case fatality for myocardial infarction were higher in deprived areas, rates of hospitalisation were lower. These findings draw attention to the ways in which patients gain initial access to care in this condition, rather than to problems of case management in hospital (see Chapter 4).

Outcomes in cancer are also worse for people living in deprived areas. Coleman *et al.* (2001) analysed cancer registry data for patients in England using the Carstairs index of the enumeration district of residence as an index of deprivation. Across a wide range of adult cancers, the five-year survival rate was 11.1 per cent lower for the most deprived subjects compared with the most affluent. Smaller differences were observed for cancers which are less amenable to treatment (lung cancer, 1 per cent difference; prostate cancer 2.9 per cent difference). Observations like these raise many questions (Coleman *et al.* 2001). Do the worse outcomes associated with lower socio-economic status result from greater severity of illness and worse general health? Can the findings be explained by reduced uptake of preventive services and delayed presentation for acute medical care? Are treatment services less accessible and the quality of care provided lower for people of lower socio-economic status? More detailed studies are needed to answer these questions. However, it is clear that health services still need to 'strive to reduce systematic disparities in health between more and less advantaged social groups' (Braveman *et al.* 2001: 679).

Vertical equity in access to health care

Vertical equity requires that groups with unequal needs are treated in proportion to their inequality. This concept is relevant when considering the needs of different socio-economic groups; it also has special relevance when considering services for different care groups. Services for older people, people with mental health problems, disabled people, or others in need of long-term care, are generally considered to be under-resourced when compared with acute services for younger adults. These are sometimes referred to as 'Cinderella services'. Cullis and West (1979) compared expenditure for patients in acute hospital beds with those in geriatric, psychiatric or mental handicap institutions. The three-fold difference in expenditure (1975–6) seemed to confirm vertical inequity favouring the acutely ill over the long-term sick and disabled. This observation was consistent with the concerns over standards of provision in long-stay institutions which were being expressed at that time.

Vertical equity is often addressed implicitly through the notions of priority setting and rationing. These concepts introduce the idea of restricting or enhancing access to health care for groups with differing needs (see Chapter 11). Concern for vertical equity also raises questions about the desirability of targeting health care delivery at groups with different needs. Targeting may be difficult to implement, may raise concerns about stigmatisation or discrimination, and targeted programmes tend to attract fewer resources than mainstream ones (Gelbach and Pritchett 2001). According to these arguments, when addressing groups with special needs it may often be more appropriate to identify and remove barriers to access to mainstream services, rather than develop new services for use by a specific group.

The related notions of priority setting, rationing and targeting were brought together in Mooney's suggestion that the benefits from health intervention (for example, the number of quality-adjusted life years gained) might be valued more highly when they accrue to groups with worse health status (Mooney, 1996). The existence of inequalities in health requires positive discrimination in the allocation and use of resources to improve the health of disadvantaged groups and reduce inequalities. A pre-occupation with horizontal equity is, Mooney argues, misplaced because this approach neutralises the fact that different groups' needs differ, and will not lead to a reduction in inequalities between groups. Thus in the UK, the formula used to allocate health care resources to different areas has been based on population size weighted for the standardised mortality ratio. This implies that it is accepted that populations with higher mortality rates should receive additional health care resources (Mooney *et al.* 2002). Work in relation to the health of indigenous Australians suggested that positive discrimination favouring a disadvantaged group with worse health would be supported by health service managers and the wider community (Mooney 2000; Wiseman and Jan 2000). However, there are obvious difficulties in adopting a quantitative approach.

The equity–efficiency trade-off

Equity and efficiency have been contrasted as policy objectives in health care (Gilson 1998). There is also a growing appreciation of the technical trade-off between equity and efficiency in the delivery of health care. An efficient health service might provide the greatest aggregated amount of access for a given level of resources, but an efficient service will not always be an equitable one because access may not be distributed fairly between groups (Williams 1997). Efforts to increase equity will often lead to a reduction in efficiency. For example, locating a specialist service in a sparsely populated rural area will improve equity of access but reduce efficiency because the service may be under-utilised. A health promotion intervention may be efficient if the majority responds to it, but inequities may be increased if it does not reach minority groups (Lindholm *et al.* 1996). These considerations lead away from a single-minded pursuit of equity, towards a recognition that inequities may only be reduced at a cost which may not always be acceptable.

Conclusions

Equity in access to health care is a recognised objective of health systems, and may be evaluated in terms of the availability, use and outcomes of health care. While there appears to be some consensus in the UK and Europe that public health care resources should be distributed equitably, the commitment to equity in health itself appears to be considerably weaker. Most studies have evaluated horizontal equity in access to health care, because there is less consensus on how the concept of vertical equity could be judged to exist.

Taking the results of generic and specific studies together, several conclusions may be drawn concerning the situation in the UK. In primary care there is evidence of inequity in the availability and structure of primary care services, with poorer areas being disadvantaged. Lower socio-economic status is generally associated with increased utilisation of primary care, but after adjusting for need there is little evidence of inequity in the utilisation of general practitioner visits. However, the type of care utilised by different groups varies with considerable inequity in the utilisation of preventive medical care. The quality of primary care received by lower socio-economic groups may also be lower. The overall utilisation of hospital services may be increased in poorer areas, but the socio-economically disadvantaged and ethnic minorities appear to gain less access to elective specialist care than the more affluent, especially if private care is taken into account (Chapter 6). Lower socio-economic status is also associated with worse health outcomes in a range of treatable conditions.

Several conclusions may be drawn from the comparison of generic and specific studies of equity in access to health care. First, conclusions may differ according to the criterion chosen to evaluate access. For example, when judged in terms of service availability and service outcomes there is considerable evidence of inequity in access to primary care services. It is only when judged according to the criterion of utilisation that a different picture emerges. Second, measures of health need should be selected which are relevant to the objectives of health care. The extent of error and bias in the assessment of health status should be specifically considered, and where possible quantified. This will be important in interpreting the results of analyses which have been adjusted for need. Third, utilisation data should be collected in such a way as to provide an insight into the content of users' contacts with services, and this information should be interpreted in relation to need.

In their review of equity and access in the UK, Goddard and Smith (1998) showed that much evidence in this area is of poor quality; they also pointed to the need to obtain new evidence in health care sectors which have been less well investigated, and to explain why inequities exist. There is also a need to evaluate the distributional consequences of new health policies and health care interventions (Sassi *et al.* 2001) (see Chapter 10). In health service planning and management, Acheson (1998) emphasised the importance of developing and promoting equity as a focus for policies in resource allocation, standard setting, quality assurance and performance management.

Turning to the question of why inequities in access to health care exist, Chapter 2 has already discussed the inevitability of geographical inequality in access to services. The influence of personal factors such as differences in help-seeking behaviour, communication difficulties and cultural preferences in treatment choices are now discussed in Chapter 4. Organisational barriers to the uptake of services for different groups are discussed in Chapter 5, while Chapters 6, 7 and 8 discuss financial barriers to access in the UK, the US and the European Union respectively. In the final chapter of the book, we discuss whether the consensus which has maintained systems such as the NHS is now being replaced by a more individualistic philosophy in which the concept of equity is regarded with different values.

References

Abasolo, I., Manning, R. and Jones, A.M. (2001) 'Equity in utilisation of and access to public sector GPs in Spain', *Applied Economics*, 33: 349–64.

Acheson, E.D. (1998) *Independent Inquiry into Inequalities in Health*. London: The Stationery Office.

Bindman, J., Glover, G., Goldberg, D. and Chisholm, D. (2000) 'Expenditure on mental health care by English health authorities: a potential cause of inequity', *British Journal of Psychiatry*, 177: 267–74.

Bommier, A. and Stecklov, G. (2002) 'Defining health inequality: why Rawls succeeds where social welfare theory fails', *Journal of Health Economics*, 21: 497–513.

Braveman, P., Starfield, B. and Geiger, H.J. (2001) 'World health report 2000: how it removes equity from the agenda for public health monitoring and policy', *British Medical Journal*, 323: 678–81.

Bunker, J.P., Frazier, H.S. and Mosteller, F. (1994) 'Improving health: measuring effects of medical care', *Milbank Quarterly*, 72: 225–58.

Campbell, S.M., Hann, M., Hacker, J., Burns, C., Oliver, D., Thapar, A., Meand, N., Safran, D.G., Roland, M.O. (2002) 'Identifying predictors of high quality care in English general practice: obervational study', *British Medical Journal*, 323: 784–7.

Carlisle, R., Groom, L.M., Avery, A.J., Boot, D. and Earwicker, S. (2000) 'Relation of out of hours activity by general practice and accident and emergency services with deprivation in Nottingham: longitudinal survey', *British Medical Journal*, 316: 520–3.

Chaturvedi, N., Rai, H., Ben Shlomo, Y. (1997) 'Lay diagnosis and health care seeking behaviour for chest pain in South Asians and Europeans', *Lancet*, 350: 1578–83.

Coleman, M.P., Babb, P., Sloggett, A., Quinn, M. and de Stavola, B. (2001) 'Socio-economic inequalities in cancer survival in England and Wales', *Cancer*, 91: 208–16.

Collins, E. and Klein, R. (1980) 'Equity and the NHS: self-reported morbidity, access and primary care', *British Medical Journal*, 281: 1111–15.

Cooper, H., Smaje, C. and Arber, S. (1998) 'Use of health services by children and young people according to ethnicity and social class: secondary analysis of a national survey', *British Medical Journal*, 317: 1047–51.

Cooper, H., Smaje, C. and Arber, S. (1999) 'Equity in health service use by children: examining the ethnic paradox', *Journal of Social Policy*, 28: 457–78.

Cullis, J.G. and West, P.A. (1979) *The economics of health. An introduction.* Oxford: Martin Robertson, 237–239.

Culyer, A.J. (1993) 'Health, health expenditures and equity'. In E. van Doorslaer, A. Wagstaff and F. Rutten (eds) *Equity in the Finance and Delivery of Health Care. An International Perspective*, pp. 299–319. Oxford: Oxford Medical Publications.

Culyer, A.J. and Wagstaff, A. (1993) 'Equity and equality in health care', *Journal of Health Economics*, 12: 431–57.

Davey Smith, G. (1997) 'Socioeconomic differentials'. In D. Kuh and Y. Ben Shlomo (eds) *A Life-course Approach to Chronic Disease Epidemiology*, pp. 242–73. Oxford: Oxford Medical Publications.

Davey Smith, G. (2000) 'Learning to live with complexity: ethnicity, socio-economic position, and health in Britain and the United States', *American Journal of Public Health*, 90: 1694–8.

Department of Health (2000) *The NHS Plan: A Plan for Investment, A Plan for Reform.* London: The Stationery Office.

Department of Health (2001a) *Quality and Performance in the NHS: High Level Performance and Clinical Indicators,* London: Department of Health. http://www.doh.gov.uk/indicat/indicat.htm; accessed 24 September 2001.

Department of Health (2001b) *Shifting the Balance*. London: Department of Health.

Dong. W., Ben Shlomo, Y., Colhoun, H., Chaturvedi, N. (1998) 'Gender differences in accessing cardiac surgery across England: a cross-sectional analysis of the Health Survey for England', *Social Science and Medicine*, 47: 1773–80.

Drever, F. and Whitehead, M. (1997) *Health Inequalities. Decennial Supplement*. Office for National Statistics. Series DS number 16. London: The Stationery Office.

Duran-Tauleria, E., Rona, R.J., Chinn, S. and Burney, P. (1996) 'Influence of ethnic group on asthma treatment in children in 1990–1: national cross sectional study', *British Medical Journal*, 313: 148–52.

Feder, G., Crook, A.M., Magee, P., Banerjee, S., Timmis, A.D., Hemingway, H. (2002) 'Ethnic differences in invasive management of coronary disease: prospective cohort study of patients undergoing angiography'. *British Medical Journal*, 324: 511–16.

Gelbach, J.B. and Pritchett, L.H. (2001) *More for the Poor is Less for the Poor: The Politics of Targeting*. Working Paper 1799. New York: World Bank.

Gillam, S.J. (1992) 'Provision of health promotion clinics in relation to population need. Another example of the inverse care law', *British Journal of General Practice*, 42: 54–6.

Gillon, R. (1986) *Philosophical Medical Ethics*, pp. 86–99. Chichester: John Wiley.

Gilson, L. (1998) 'Discussion. In defence and pursuit of equity', *Social Science and Medicine*, 47: 1891–6.

Goddard, M. and Smith, P. (1998) *Equity of Access to Health Care*. York: University of York, Centre for Health Economics.

Goddard, M. and Smith, P. (2001) 'Equity of access to health care services: theory and evidence from the UK', *Social Science and Medicine*, 53: 1149–62.

Gravelle, H. and Sutton, M. (2001) 'Inequality in the geographical distribution of general practitioners in England and Wales 1974–95', *Journal of Health Service Research Policy*, 6: 6–13.

Gulliford, M.C. (2002) 'Availability of primary care doctors and population health in England: is there an association?', *Journal of Public Health Medicine*, 24: 252–4.

Gulliford, M.C. and Mahabir, D. (2001) 'Utilisation of private care by public primary care clinic attenders with diabetes: relationship to health status and social factors', *Social Science and Medicine*', 53: 1045–56.

Gutmann, A. (1981) 'For and against equal access in health care', *Milbank Memorial Fund Quarterly*, 59: 542–60.

Haynes, R. (1991) 'Inequalities in health and health service use: evidence from the General Household Survey', *Social Science and Medicine*, 33: 361–8.

Hippisley-Cox, J. and Pringle, M. (2000) 'Inequalities in access to coronary angiography and revascularisation: the association of deprivation and location of primary care services', *British Journal of General Practice*, 50: 449–54.

Hull, S.A., Tissier, J., Moser, K., Derrett, C.J., Carter, Y.H. and Eldridge, S. (2000) 'Lessons from the London Initiative Zone Educational Incentives funding: associations between practice characteristics, funding and courses undertaken', *British Journal of General Practice*, 50: 183–7.

Judge, K.and Mays, N. (1994). 'Equity in the NHS. Allocating resources for health and social care in England', *British Medical Journal*, 308: 1363–6.

Khunti, K., Ganguli, S. and Lowy, A. (2001) 'Inequalities in provision of systematic care for patients with diabetes', *Family Practice*, 18: 27–32.

Kunst, A.E., Groenhof, F., Mackenbach, J.P. and the EU Working Group on socio-economic inequalities in health (1998) 'Occupational class and cause specific mortality in middle aged men in 11 European countries: comparison of population based studies', *British Medical Journal*, 316: 1636–42.

Lang, T., Ducimetiere, P., Arvelier, D., Amouyel, P., Ferrieres, J., Ruidavets, J.B., Monatye, M., Haas, B. and Bingham, A. (1998) 'Is hospital care involved in inequalities in coronary heart disease mortality? Results from the French WHO MONICA project in men aged 30 to 64 years', *Journal of Epidemiology Community Health*, 52: 665–71.

Leese, B. and Bosanquet, N. (1995) 'Change in general practice and its effects on service provision in areas with different socio-economic characteristics', *British Medical Journal*, 311: 546–50.

Le Grand, J. (1978). 'The distribution of public expenditure. The case of health care', *Economica*, 45: 125–42.

Lindholm, L., Rosen, M. and Emmelin, M. (1996) 'An epidemiological approach towards measuring the trade off between equity and efficiency in health policy', *Health Policy*, 35: 205–16.

Lorant, V., Boland, B., Humblet, P. and Deliege, D. (2002) 'Equity in prevention and health care', *Journal of Epidemiology and Community Health*, 56: 510–16.

Lynch, M. (1995) 'Effect of practice and patient population characteristics on the uptake of childhood immunisations', *British Journal of General Practice*, 45: 205–8.

Macintyre, S., Ellaway, A. and Cummins, S. (2002) 'Place effects on health: how can we conceptualise, operationalise and measure them?', *Social Science and Medicine*, 55: 125–39.

Mackenbach, J.P. and Kunst, A.E. (1997) 'Measuring the magnitude of socio-economic inequalities in health: An overview of available measures illustrated with two examples from Europe', *Social Science and Medicine*, 44: 757–71.

Majeed, F.A., Cook, D.G., Anderson, H.R., Hilton, S., Bunn, S. and Stones, C. (1994) 'Using patient and general practice characteristics to explain variations in cervical smear uptake rates', *British Medical Journal*, 308: 1272–6.

Manor, O., Matthews, S. and Power, C. (1997) 'Comparing measures of health inequality', *Social Science and Medicine*, 45: 761–71.

McIntyre, D. and Gilson, L. (2000). 'Redressing disadvantage: Promoting vertical equity within South Africa', *Health Care Analysis* 8: 235–58.

Mooney, G. (1996) 'And now for vertical equity? Some concerns arising from Aboriginal health in Australia', *Health Economics*, 5: 99–103.

Mooney, G. (2000) 'Vertical equity in health care resource allocation', *Health Care Analysis*, 8: 203–15.

Mooney, G., Jan, S. and Wideman, V. (2002) 'Staking a claim for claims: a case study of resource allocation in Australian Aboriginal health care', *Social Science and Medicine*, 54: 1657–67.

Morrison, C., Woodward, M., Leslie, W. and Tunstall-Pedoe, H. (1997) 'Effect of socio-economic group on incidence of, management of, and survival after myocardial infarction and coronary death: analysis of community coronary event register', *British Medical Journal*, 314: 541–6.

Murray, C.J.L. (2001) 'Commentary: comprehensive approaches are needed for full understanding', *British Medical Journal*, 323: 678–81.

O'Donnell, O. and Propper, C. (1991) 'Equity and the distribution of UK National Health Service resources', *Journal for Health Economics*, 10: 1–19.

Pan American Health Organisation (2001) 'Measuring health inequalities: Gini coefficient and concentration index', *Epidemiological Bulletin*, 22: 3–4.

Paterson, I. and Judge, K. (2002). 'Equality of access to health care'. In J. Mackenbach and M. Bakker (eds) *Reducing Inequalities in Health: A European Perspective*. London: Routledge.

Payne, N. and Saul, C. (1997) 'Variations in use of cardiology services in a health authority: comparison of coronary artery revascularisation rates with prevalence of angina and coronary mortality', *British Medical Journal*, 314: 257–61.

Pell, J.P., Pell, A.C.H., Norrie, J., Ford, I. and Cobbe, S.M. (2000) 'Effect of socio-economic deprivation on waiting time for cardiac surgery: retrospective cohort study, *British Medical Journal*, 320: 15–19.

Powell, M. (1992) 'Hospital provision before the NHS: territorial justice or inverse care law?', *Journal for Social Policy*, 21: 145–63.

Puffer, F. (1986) 'Access to primary health care: a comparison of the US and the UK', *Journal for Social Policy*, 15: 293–313.

Raine, R. (2000) 'Does gender bias exist in the use of specialist care?', *Journal for Health Services Research Policy*, 5: 237–49.

Rawls, J. (1999) *A Theory of Justice*. Oxford: Oxford University Press.

Reinhardt, U. (1996) 'A social contract for 21st century health care: three tier health care with bounty hunting', *Health Economics*, 5: 479–500.

Salisbury, C., Trivella, M. and Bruster, S. (2000) 'Demand for and supply of out of hours care from general practitioners in England and Scotland: observational study based on routinely collected data', *British Medical Journal*, 320: 618–21.

Sassi, F., Archard, L. and Le Grand, J. (2001) 'Equity and the economic evaluation of health care', *Health Technology Assessment*, 5(3): 1–138.

Seddon, M.E., Marshall, M.N., Campbell, S.M. and Roland, M.O. (2001) 'Systematic review of studies of quality of clinical care in general practice in the UK, Australia and New Zealand', *Quality of Health Care*, 10: 152–8.

Shi, L. and Starfield, B. (2001) 'The effect of primary care physician supply and income inequality on mortality among blacks and whites in US Metropolitan areas', *American Journal of Public Health*, 91: 1246–50.

Shi, L., Starfield, B., Kennedy, B. and Kawachi, I. (1999) 'Income inequality, primary care, and health indicators', *Journal of Family Practice*, 48: 275–84.

Smaje, C. (1995) *Health, Race and Ethnicity. Making Sense of the Evidence*. London: King's Fund Institute.

Smaje, C. and Le Grand, J. (1997) 'Ethnicity equity and the use of health services in the British NHS', *Social Science and Medicine*, 45: 485–96.

Smith, P., Sheldon, T.A., Carr-Hill, R.A., Martin, S., Peacock, S. and Hardman G. (1994) 'Allocating resources to health authorities: results and policy implications of small area analysis of use of inpatient services', *British Medical Journal*, 309: 1050–4.

Stevens, A. and Raftery, J. (1994) 'Introduction'. In A. Stevens and J. Raftery (eds) *Health Care Needs Assessment. The Epidemiologically Based Needs Assessment Reviews*, pp. 11–28. Oxford: Radcliffe Medical.

Stirling, A.M., Wilson, P. and McConnachie, A. (2001) 'Deprivation, psychological distress and consultation length in general practice', *British Journal of General Practice*, 51: 456–60.

Sutton, M., Carr-Hill, R., Gravelle, H. and Rice, N. (1999) 'Do measures of self-reported morbidity bias the estimation of the determinants of health care utilisation?', *Social Science and Medicine*, 49: 867–78.

Szwarcwald, C.L. (2002) 'On the World Health Organisation's measurement of health inequalities', *Journal of Epidemiology and Community Health*, 56: 177–82.

Tudor Hart, J. (1971) 'The inverse care law', *Lancet*, 7696: 405–12.

Tudor Hart, J. (2001) 'Three decades of the inverse care law', *British Medical Journal* 320: 15–19.

van Doorslaer, E., Koolman X. and Puffer, F. (2002) 'Equity in the use of physician visits in OECD countries: has equal treatment for equal need been achieved?'. In P. Smith (ed.) *Measuring Up: Improving Health System Performance in OECD Countries*, 225–48. Paris: Organisation for Economic Co-operation and Development.

van Doorslaer, E., Wagstaff, A. and Rutten, F. (1993) *Equity in the Finance and Delivery of Health Care. An International Perspective*. Oxford: Oxford Medical Publications.

van Doorslaer, E., Wagstaff, A., van der Burg, Christiansen, T., de Graeve, D. and Duchesne, I. *et al.* (2000) 'Equity in the delivery of health care in Europe and the US', *Journal of Health Economics*, 19: 553–83.

Wagstaff, A., Paci, P. and van Doorslaer, E. (1991a) 'On the measurement of inequalities in health', *Social Science and Medicine*, 33: 545–57.

Wagstaff, A., van Doorslaer, E. and Paci, P. (1991) 'On the measurement of horizontal inequity in the delivery of health care', *Journal of Health Economics*, 10: 169–205.

Wagstaff, A., van Doorslaer, E., van der Burg, H., Calonge, S., Christiansen, T. and Citoni, G., Gerdtham, U.G., Gerfin, M., Gross, L., Hakkinen, U., Johnson, P. John, J., Klavus, J., Lachaud, C., Lauritsen, J., Leu, R., Nolan, B., Peran, E., Pereira, J., Propper, C., Puffer, F., Rochaix, L., Rodriguez, M., Schellhorn, M. and Winkelhake, O. (1999) 'Equity in the finance of health care: some further international comparisons', *Journal of Health Economics*, 18: 263–90.

Whitehead, M., Evandrou, M., Haglund, B. and Diderichsen, F. (1997) 'As the health divide widens in Sweden and Britain, what's happening to access to care?', *British Medical Journal*, 315: 1006–9.

Williams, A. (1993) 'Equity in health care: the role of ideology'. In E. van Doorslaer, A. Wagstaff and F. Rutten (eds) *Equity in the Finance and Delivery of Health Care. An International Perspective*, pp. 287–98. Oxford: Oxford Medical Publications.

Williams, A. (1997) 'Intergenerational equity: an exploration of the fair innings argument', *Health Economics*, 6: 117–32.

Wiseman, V. and Jan, S. (2000) 'Resource allocation within Australian indigenous communities: a programme for implementing vertical equity', *Health Care Analysis*, 8: 217–233.

World Health Organisation (2000) *The World Health Report 2000*. Geneva: World Health Organisation.

Chapter 4

Patients' help-seeking and access to health care

Myfanwy Morgan

Introduction

Access to health care requires both that the population has access in terms of the availability of services and that people take the steps necessary to gain access. Individual behaviours thus form a key determinant of whether and when services are utilised but patient behaviours often do not conform to medical or managerial expectations of appropriate and timely service use. This chapter first examines what have traditionally been regarded as the twin 'problems' of patients' delay or non-uptake of services and their inappropriate use of services. It then discusses four types of explanations and models developed to account for these patient behaviours. These are individualistic approaches, social barriers explanations, patient-oriented approaches and a social strategy approach. The chapter concludes with a discusssion of changing policy assumptions and service configurations that place greater emphasis on enabling access through diverse sources to meet patients' needs.

Patients' uptake of services

In the UK the process of accessing medical services (except in emergencies), has traditionally involved a single route of presenting to a general practitioner, who serves as the initial point of contact for 90 per cent of NHS consultations and the gatekeeper to hospital services for non-emergency conditions. Patients' initial behaviour in accessing health care and particularly seeking a GP consultation thus largely determines whether and when diagnosis and treatment occur and influences receipt of both primary and hospital services.

Problems of delay and non-uptake

Surveys conducted in the UK and other countries from the 1950s onwards indicated that the experience of symptoms was common but only a minority were brought to professional medical attention, even where, as in the NHS, health services are free at the point of use. Instead much illness was ignored, or managed through self-medication or other self-care, and was described as comprising an 'iceberg' of untreated illness in the community (Koos 1954; Wadsworth *et al.* 1971; Hannay 1979; Van der Lisdonk 1989; Kookier 1995). As might be expected, the rate of professional-help-seeking is greater for more serious conditions than for minor ailments. However, there was evidence of a considerable 'clinical iceberg' (a subset of the 'iceberg of illness') comprising more serious conditions that did not receive professional medical attention, or experienced considerable delays in medical care contact (Last 1963). As Mechanic (1962) observed, 'Such considerations lead us to propose a concept of *illness behaviour*. By this term we refer to the ways in which given symptoms may be differentially perceived, evaluated and acted (or not acted) upon by different kinds of persons' (p. 189). Mechanic thus identified two aspects of patients' professional-help-seeking: the evaluation of symptoms and the decision concerning the appropriate course of action.

Despite many changes in health service provision and patterns of service use over the past 30 years, there is still evidence that much illness is managed through self-care. For example, Rogers and colleagues (1999) found in a household based study using four-week health diaries that no health action was reported for 24 per cent of illness episodes, only self-care activities were reported for 54 per cent, self-care activities and professional health care were reported for 17 per cent of illness episodes and only professional care was reported for about 5 per cent of illness episodes. There are also continuing concerns about patients' failure to gain appropriate and timely access to both acute and preventive health services. For example, although there has been a notable increase in the coverage of preventive services, recent figures indicate that 16 per cent of women aged 25–64 years resident in England had not received cervical screening at least once in the previous five years (Department of Health 2000a). For mammography, 32 per cent of women aged 50–64 resident in England and 26 per cent for women aged 55–64 years had not attended for x-ray mammography at least once in the previous three years (Department of Health 2000b). Despite a trend toward increasing rates of childhood immunisation, recent parental concerns about the triple MMR (measles, mumps and rubella) vaccine has resulted in a decline in uptake at 24 months in England to 84 per cent, which is some way off the recommended target of 95 per cent (Communicable Disease Surveillance Centre 2001). A general finding is that people from the poorer socio-economic groups with the greatest morbidity and hence needs for services (and populations in deprived areas) have the lowest rates of uptake of a range of preventive services, including rates of uptake of cervical screening, mammography and childhood immunisations (Lynch 1995; Reading *et al.* 1994). Differences in uptake may also be greater for more recent forms of screening such as cholesterol testing (Chapter 3).

Some subgroups experience particular problems in accessing services. For example, women with learning difficulties have particularly low rates of uptake of cervical screening in the UK and it is suspected that studies of other treatments and preventive interventions might find the same (Smith 1999). Patterns of uptake of preventive services by ethnic group are also mixed. The uptake of childhood immunisations is generally higher among the main ethnic minority groups in the UK (particularly South Asian) compared with the white population, but several studies indicate that rates of uptake of breast and cervical screening are relatively low among South Asian women in the UK. There is also evidence of local variations, which may reflect differences in the socio-economic status and other characteristics of ethnic groups in different areas (Atkinson *et al.* 2001).

For acute services there are concerns about delays in uptake for conditions that benefit from early detection and treatment. For example, it is well established that rapid thrombolysis can limit damage following myocardial infarction and reduce risk of death, but there is considerable patient delay in medical care contact, often compounded by further medical and health service related delay. A study in six district hospitals in England found that patients with coronary symptoms took a median time of 40 minutes to call the emergency services and 70 minutes to call their general practitioner. The median time from call to arrival in hospital was 41 minutes for patients who called an ambulance from home and 90 minutes for people who contacted their doctor (Birkhead 1992). Data from the Glasgow MONICA project also showed that only 25 per cent of surviving cases of myo-cardial infarction made a call for help within one hour of the onset of coronary symptoms, and for 40 per cent the delay was greater than four hours (Leslie *et al.* 2000). Breast cancer is another condition for which there is concern about the adverse effect of delays, with evidence that five-year survival rates are 12 per cent lower among women whose breast cancer treatment does not begin until three months or more after their first symptoms appear. Studies in the UK indicate that between 20 per cent and 30 per cent of women who detect a breast lump do not visit the doctor until three months or more have elapsed, and subsequent service-related delay then frequently occurs prior to the first hospital appointment (Jones 1999). Significant delays have been documented in relation to patients' uptake of services for a range of other non-infectious conditions, including dyspepsia (Delaney 1998), glaucoma (Fraser *et al.* 2001) and mental illness (Shaw *et al.* 1999), and a number of communicable and infectious diseases including sexually transmitted diseases (Meyer-Weitz *et al.* 2000) and lower urinary tract symptoms (Shaw *et al.* 2001).

Socio-economically disadvantaged groups frequently exhibit the greatest delays in contacting medical services for diagnosis and treatment. Typical socio-economic risk factors were identified by a study of late presentation of advanced glaucoma based on three eye departments in England, with late presenters being predomi-nately from areas with higher median underprivileged area scores, of lower social class, more likely to have no access to a car and to be tenants rather than owner occupiers, and including a high proportion of African Caribbean people (Fraser *et al.* 2001). Lower socio-economic occupational position and social deprivation has also been linked to later presentation of a variety of other conditions including cancers (Wells and Horm 1992; Robinson *et al.* 1995). Rates of GP consultations among the main ethnic groups appear to be comparable with the general population, but are lower for some groups including Chinese, Africans and young Pakistanis

(Goddard and Smith 2001). Other disadvantaged groups with low rates of uptake of GP services are homeless people who comprise a heterogeneous population and include young employed men sleeping on the streets, mentally ill people, drug addicts and others sleeping rough or in hostels. Despite high morbidity rates, homeless people are more likely to delay accessing services and present with disease rather than at the preventive and screening stages. A survey of residents of a residential centre for homeless people in London found that many had physical illnesses but three-fifths had not seen a GP for more than five years (Crane and Warnes 2001). Low uptake of GP services is associated with low rates of registration with a GP and a tendency to rely on accident and emergency (A&E) departments for primary care (Plearce and Quilgares 1996; Power *et al.* 1999). Other groups with inappropriately low rates uptake of health services are traveller gypsies and new refugee groups who in the UK currently include people from Afghanistan, Sri Lanka, Somalia and Kosovo. In 1997 new refugees were estimated to comprise a population of 230,000 of whom over half lived in London. Many GPs are reluctant to accept these groups on to their lists due to problems of paperwork, concerns about demands of care and, in the case of new refugee groups, concerns about patients' eligibility for services (Jones and Gill 1998).

The emphasis of utilisation studies is on patients' initial contacts with medical care, but patients may also encounter other barriers to their progress through the system. For example, there is some evidence that socio-economically disadvantaged groups and some ethnic minorities may have reduced access to specialist services, associated with local variations in service availability and individual clinical decisions (Payne and Saul 1997; Feder *et al.* 2002). Data also show considerable patient non-attendance for booked appointments, with 12 per cent non-attendance for hospital outpatient appointments in the UK and considerable variation between specialties and regions. Figures for non-attendance for GP appointments range from 3 per cent to 6.5 per cent (Sharp and Hamilton 2001). Non-attendance has been identified as a particular problem in deprived areas (Neal *et al.* 2001). There are also concerns that non-attenders at psychiatric outpatient clinics are often more severely ill and difficult to engage (Killaspy *et al.* 1999).

Problems of 'over-utilisation'

Whereas one set of concerns relates to patient delays and non-uptake of services, a second set relates to what has been defined as patients' 'inappropriate' use of services. At a primary care level GPs frequently complain that patients consult inappropriately with medical 'trivia', and 'frequent attenders' are regarded as making unnecessary demands on services (Heywood *et al.* 1998). Frequent attenders are varyingly defined as patients who attend more than seven, eight or twelve times a year, or who form the upper 10 per cent of consulting frequency. They are mainly drawn from poorer sections of the population, and tend to be female, living alone and living in urban areas, and attend with a high level of non-specific complaints and mental health problems (Heywood *et al.* 1998; Jiwa 2000). The designation of patients as making 'inappropriate' demands on services is influenced by medical professionals' expertise and views of their appropriate role, with more experienced doctors often being less likely to perceive patients as 'difficult'. General practitioners whose style of practice emphasises the social and psychological dimensions of illness also define a higher proportion of consultations as requiring professional attention and therefore as 'necessary' (Steinmetz and Tabenkin, 2001; Morgan 2003).

Other concerns relate to the substantial increase in demands on out-of-hours primary care services in the UK. Actions in response to out-of-hours calls identify varying needs. However, studies indicate that between 41 per cent and 60 per cent of out-of-hours contacts in primary care are considered 'inappropriate' (Hallam 1994). Out-of-hours primary care is now increasingly provided through patients calling deputising services or attending primary care centres rather than by home visits. However, the growth of primary care centres raises questions of their accessibility to deprived populations, especially late at night or for people with young children (Shipman *et al.* 2001).

The appropriateness of patient demands has formed a continuing concern in relation to hospital A&E departments. Surveys define large numbers of A&E attenders as neither accidents nor emergencies, relatively few of whom require specific hospital treatment. The British Association of Accident and Emergency Medicine classified between 10 per cent and 40 per cent of A&E attenders as needing primary care rather than A&E services (National Audit Office 1992). Other reviews provide a greater range; from 6 per cent to 80 per cent of A&E attenders have been classified as 'inappropriate' in the UK, and international figures suggest 7–70 per cent (Robertson-Steel 1998). The proportion of new A&E attendees with primary care problems tends to be much lower in more affluent areas compared with deprived populations and inner city hospitals (Carlisle *et al.* 1998; Murphy 1998a). Differences in the characteristics of local populations do not however entirely explain the varying proportions of patients classified as inappropriate users of A&E services by different studies, with this also reflecting the lack of professional consensus regarding 'appropriate' attenders and what constitutes an 'emergency'. 'Appropriate' attendance may be narrowly defined according to the clinical severity of the illness, or defined more broadly to take account of the social circumstances under which the illness occurs, whether the accident or injury occurred outside normal general practice hours, and the psychological responses of the patient and their family in terms of their anxiety, fears and distress (Calnan 1982). Variations in professional views of appropriate attendance have been attributed to differences in professional training, speciality, frustration with minor ailment management, and the perceived availability of other services and sources of advice (Morris *et al.* 2001). Questions of the nature and determinants of medical and administrative definitions of appropriate uptake of services have received relatively little attention, while patients' help-seeking behaviour has formed a major focus of research.

This section has identified the importance of patient behaviours in determining whether and when services are accessed and has presented some evidence from the large literature documenting variations in help-seeking behaviours among social groups (for detailed reviews see Goddard and Smith 2001; Atkinson *et al.* 2001). The next section examines explanations for patients' help-seeking behaviours. Although much help-seeking involves the use of over-the-counter medicines and the use of complementary medicines and practitioners, this chapter focuses particularly on the uptake of formal medical services and reasons for the divergence in patient behaviours from professional expectations of service use.

Explaining patients' help-seeking

Explanations of professional help-seeking and use of services can be classified into the four broad groups based on their main emphasis and explanatory framework. These are: individualistic approaches, social barriers approaches, patient-oriented approaches, and a social strategy approach.

Individualistic approaches

Both individualistic and social barriers approaches adopt medical definitions of appropriate patient behaviour and attempt to explain non-conformity with professional expectations by comparing users and non-users on factors hypothesised to influence patients' uptake of services. Individualistic approaches derive from social-psychological research and focus on individuals' attributes as encouraging or discouraging professional-help-seeking. Social-psychological models of patient behaviours mainly consist of structured cognition models that attempt to identify cognitive processes underlying decision-making. Examples are the protection motivation theory (Rogers 1975) that regards motivation to engage in some kind of health protective behaviour as depending on the perceived severity of the disease, the perceived probability of its occurrence and the efficacy of the recommended response. The theory of reasoned behaviour (Ajzen and Fishbein 1980) also depicts behavioural intentions as the product of people's beliefs and evaluations regarding the outcome of the behaviour, the normative beliefs of family and friends and motivation to comply with these beliefs. These and other social cognition models contributed to the multifactoral Health Belief Model (HMB) originally put forward by Rosenstock (1966). The HBM was derived from social-psychological learning theory and aimed to explain why people failed to make use of disease prevention or screening tests for the early detection of disease. The original model has since undergone a number of modifications and is now applied to both preventive health behaviours and the uptake of medical services in response to symptoms (Rosenstock 1974; Becker and Maiman 1975; Becker *et al.* 1977). The HBM assumes that an individual's readiness to engage in a given health behaviour is the outcome of a rational cost–benefit analysis that depends on four groups of factors: 1) the perceived threat of the disease, which depends on beliefs about their own susceptibility to the disease and its severity; 2) the perceived benefits of a particular course of action; 3) perceived barriers to seeking care (e.g. transport costs, lost time from work, side effects of drugs); 4) the influence of an individual's general health motivation or readiness to be concerned about health matters. Perceptions and actions are also now presented as affected by internal cues (e.g. pain) and external cues (e.g. influence of mass media). These dimensions are also influenced by demographic variables (age, class, gender, etc.) and by psychological character-istics (personality, peer group pressure, etc.).

The HBM has been employed to predict and explain behaviour in a variety of settings, including GP consultation behaviour (Campbell and Roland 1996; Van der Kar et al. 1992), the use of accident and emergency services (Walsh 1995), and the uptake of preventive services (Calnan 1984; Gillam 1991). The HBM has provided a useful framework for research and identified the importance of specific dimensions (e.g. perceived susceptibility, severity, benefits and barriers) in relation to the uptake of a range of preventive and medical services (Janz and Becker 1984; Harrison et al. 1992). A limitation of research deriving from the HBM is that its variables are operationalised in different ways in different studies, which reduces possibilities for comparison. The HBM has also been found to explain only a small amount of the total variance in behaviours between defaulters and appropriate service users, possibly reflecting the relative insensitivity of measures that do not gauge the meanings attributed by individuals to cues or other factors.

Andersen's (1968) Social Behavioural Model (SBM) is a multi-factor model that like the HBM was developed in the 1960s. It was initially presented as a behavioural model to explain how families use health services (Andersen and Newman 1973; Andersen 1995) but can be classified as a social barriers model in terms of its emphasis on structural factors that impede the take-up of services. The SBM has also undergone substantial modifications and now closely parallels the HBM, although remaining more structurally oriented and emphasising income and health insurance as enabling factors. Criticisms of the SBM are similar to those of the HBM. Both assume that the main motivation and determinant of preventive health behaviours and conformity with health promotion advice is individuals' desire for long-term health gain, whereas short-term contingencies may often be more influential. They are also concerned exclusively with the use of professional medical care rather than taking account of the range of alternative health actions. New developments in social-psychological research aim to respond to these limitations by expanding their focus and often distinguish between spontaneous and deliberate behaviours (Conner and Norman 1996).

Social barriers approaches

This refers to explanations for patients' non-conformity with medical expectations and definitions of appropriate behaviours in terms of social and situational forces that impinge on individuals and social groups and prompt or delay professional-help-seeking. Four main types of factors deriving from different disciplinary perspectives have been identified as barriers (or factors that facilitate) service use. These are:

Economic factors

Specific economic factors identified as relevant for transforming need into demand include income, health insurance cover, travel costs, the costs of health services and the availability of free medical care. These factors have their greatest influence in systems where co-payments are required and among the poorest sections of the population with least command of economic resources (see Chapters 6 and 8).

Geographic factors

These place particular emphasis on the proximity of services and travel times as determinants of individuals' utilisation. A number of studies show that increasing distance is associated with lower use of services, including the uptake of screening and immunisation (Goddard and Smith 2001), primary care (Nemet and Bailey 2000), and A&E services (Campbell 1994). However, although distance from the service, and especially the travel time and costs involved, are a deterrent, these effects depend on the nature of the service and have a greater effect on emergency than on elective admissions. They also have their greatest impact on elderly and disabled patients and those with transport difficulties in rural areas (Haynes 1991) (see Chapter 2).

Organisational and medical care factors

This focuses on the effects of health care organisation and the experience of health care for service utilisation. For example, organisational factors that contribute to individuals' non-uptake (or delayed uptake) of primary care include problems relating to opening times, waiting times and appointment systems, patients' previous experience of medical care, and the quality of doctor–patient relationship. Other barriers or inducements relate to specific services and include the effects on the uptake of mammography and cervical screening of the known availability of a female doctor, the accessibility of services, and a well-organised system of recall and follow up of non-attenders (Yabroff and Mandelblatt 1999). Reasons for presenting at A&E services inappropriately similarly include long delays in seeing a GP, the likelihood of a subsequent referral to hospital, mistrust of the GP or lack of confidence in their ability to treat, perceptions of the relative roles of GPs and hospital doctors, proximity and ease of access to A&E, and the difficulties of seeing a GP out of hours (Prince and Worth 1992; Nguyen-Van-Tam 1992; Hallam 1994; Green and Dale 1992; Campbell 1994). Patients' prior experience with medical care and relationships with the doctor also feeds back into how illnesses are subsequently managed. This includes a sense of what the doctor considers to be a legitimate illness and the way that illness is responded to by health professionals (Rogers et al. 1999).

Medical care barriers are identified as of particular significance for populations in deprived areas, reflecting what Tudor Hart (1971) originally described as the 'inverse care law'. This refers to a situation in which the most socially deprived groups with the greatest morbidity and health needs have the least access to primary care services and attend surgeries with poorer premises and facilities (see Chapter 2). Special problems can also arise in the use of services for some ethnic minority groups. For example, low rates of uptake of GP out-of-hours services (and higher rates of A&E attendance) may reflect a lack of knowledge of out-of-hours services, difficulty using answering services and being unaware of out-of-hours interpreter arrangements (Free *et al.* 1999). Marginalised groups including alcoholics, drug addicts, traveller gypsies, the mentally ill and single homeless people are also generally poorly served by GP services and sometimes 'excluded' due to their transient lifestyle, high treatment needs and poor compliance (Crane and Warnes 2001).

Issues of the organisation and availability of services also have particular significance for people residing in institutional accommodation. A small-scale survey based on telephone interviews with 12 residential homes for elderly people indicated that individual homes often deal with four or five GPs. Regular clinics were held in some homes (usually weekly) open only to patients of the GP organising the clinic. For other residents, GPs visited only when asked to do by home staff and some homes reported difficulties in getting GPs to visit residents, especially as few homes pay extra money to GPs for the care of their residents (Kavanagh and Knapp 1998, 1999). Arrangements thus appeared to be fairly ad hoc with considerable within-home variation in individual arrangements for primary care and in opportunities for gaining access to GP services.

Prisoners form another institutional group with particular needs for health services but special barriers to access. Common health problems of prison populations are high rates of mental illness, including depression, functional psychosis and personality disorder, high rates of transmission of blood borne viruses (HIV, hepatitis C and B), and high rates of chronic physical conditions such as asthma, epilepsy and diabetes (Reed and Lyne 2000). In the UK, prisons were not incorporated into the NHS in 1948 and are still not fully, although a five-year transfer process is proposed. The governor of each prison is responsible for the prison health service and staff and allocates money from the total prison budget for health care. A review of 19 prisons in England and Wales, 1996-97, identified few prisons as providing a quality of care close to that in the NHS. Services for mentally ill prisoners have been found to fall far below standards in the NHS, with severe restrictions in both patients' ability to access services and the quality of treatment and care provided (Reed and Lyne 1997). A recent report by a joint Prison Service and NHS Executive working group (1999) endorsed the recommendation that prison health care should aim to give prisoners access to the same quality and range of health care services as the general public receives from the NHS, and recommended a formal partnership between the prison service and the NHS.

Knowledge, beliefs and roles

Low educational levels and lack of knowledge about the availability and benefits of service use are identified as factors contributing to a low uptake of preventive services among socio-economically disadvantaged groups. It has been hypothesised that the low uptake of preventive services by poorer groups may reflect a distinctive set of cultural attitudes characterised by a lack of control of one's life and a sense of fatalism that reduces the value given to long-term preventive actions. However, short-termist and fatalistic attitudes are now generally regarded as a response to structural conditions that offer the poorest groups little control over their lives, rather than forming a cultural attitude that is transmitted across generations (Naish 1994).

Social barriers approaches have been important in identifying factors that impede service use or influence the choice of service, with the number and impacts of barriers being greatest for groups characterised as having low incomes, low educational levels and high rates of unemployment, and for recent migrants from different cultural backgrounds, as well as for institutional populations. These findings have focused on the importance of reducing barriers and facilitating access for disadvantaged populations and underpinned policies to achieve greater geographical equity of health service provision (Chapter 2) and to remove financial barriers to service use in market-oriented health systems (see Cooper *et al.* 2002 for a review of approaches to reducing barriers to service use).

Patient-oriented approaches

This approach derives from an interpretive perspective that portrays individuals as conscious, reflective actors engaged in a process of making sense of their social worlds. It therefore accepts the existence of a fundamental difference between *disease* as a pathological condition and the individual's experience of *illness* in the context of their everyday lives. Individuals are thus depicted as making sense of various types of body changes within the framework of his or her own 'lay' knowledge, rather than responding in fairly predictable ways to social influences. This has led to an important shift in the questions addressed, with greater emphasis placed on such questions as: how do people define health? How do people assess their health risks? How do they identify and explain illness? And what do they do about it? The latter includes courses of action adopted prior to or instead of consulting the doctor, including self-medication, consulting pharmacists, and the use of complementary remedies and practitioners, which now have a large and specialised literature (Rogers *et al.* 1999). These issues have generally been examined, at least initially, through qualitative methods using semi-structured interviews or focus groups to elicit patients' own perspectives and the reasons for their actions rather than being required to respond to pre-defined questions with fixed-choice response categories. However, qualitative research may be followed by quantitative survey research to establish the prevalence of particular dimensions and variables identified by respondents (Barbour 1999).

A major focus of qualitative research has been the content of lay health beliefs and theories of illness and their influence on interpretations and responses to symptoms. This has included detailed studies of how lay people define health and their beliefs about the causes of illness. An important finding is the prevalence of a functional definition of health (health as the ability to undertake everyday activities), which is especially common among elderly people and more disadvantaged populations. This definition of health may contribute to delays in professional-help-seeking, with professional medical care contact not regarded as necessary until ill health severely impedes everyday activities. In terms of the uptake of preventive services and responses to health promotion messages it has also been found that lay people often make assessments about whether they feel personally vulnerable to a particular disease and act accordingly. For example, cancer is frequently identified as a disease people fear and dread getting, but individuals do not always feel personally vulnerable, reflecting notions of the importance of hereditary risks (Calnan and Johnson 1985). Similarly, there are well developed lay views of what sort of people are 'candidates' for heart trouble, based on physical appearance, the existence of heart trouble within the family, the geographical area of residence and type of work, and personal behaviours in terms of diet, smoking and worry. This information is then drawn on by lay people in responding to health promotion advice and preventive measures, and interpreting and acting in relation to symptoms (Davison *et al.* 1991).

Respondents' own accounts of help-seeking behaviours often describe their experience of considerable uncertainty about the seriousness and possible effects of symptoms. In some situations this leads to a consultation or attendance at an A&E department. An example is Roberts' (1992) in-depth study of parents' use of an A&E department in a children's hospital. This indicated that A&E attendance for relatively minor conditions often occurred when parents found it difficult to predict the outcome of an illness but were worried about failing to recognise a serious problem, and were concerned to act responsibly and protect their child. Kai (1996) described similar reasons for parents deciding to consult their GP about childhood cough. Although such actions can be viewed as rational from the parents' perspective they may result in high levels of consultation for so called medical 'trivia'. There is some evidence that in the UK grandmothers may have a beneficial role in providing reassurance for families with young children and reducing use of A&E services, although this relationship has not been demonstrated in the US (Fergusson *et al.* 1998).

Whereas one response to uncertainty is to seek professional help, in other situations uncertainty may lead to inappropriate delays in professional-help-seeking, especially if accompanied by a lack of knowledge of treatment options, embarrassment and fear of invasive investigations (Shaw *et al.* 2001). A study of responses to chest pain showed that a widely held stereotypical image of people with heart attacks collapsing with crushing chest pains did not accord with the realities for many patients. As a result a large number of people did not realise that their symptoms were coronary in origin, which led to extended delay in calling an ambulance. Non-delayers were identified as being more likely to know about other symptoms such as sweating, nausea and pains in the arm and neck (Ruston *et al.* 2000). Another source of uncertainty arises for people with multiple conditions due to the problem of distinguishing particular symptoms (such as symptoms of heart disease) from other symptoms and morbidities. Richards and colleagues observed that people from deprived areas experienced greater uncertainty and difficulty in identifying chest pain as a symptom of heart disease because they had greater exposure to ill health. This allowed them to normalise chest pain and also led to more problems in separating symptoms of heart problems from other conditions, thus extending delay in presentation. A comparison of the reporting of chest pain by men and women also indicated that the greater known risk of heart disease among men was associated with greater reporting, whereas greater uncertainty for women led to more concerns about wasting the doctor's time (Richards *et al.* 2002).

There is a general relationship between people's accurate knowledge of symptoms and service use. However, this relationship is often mediated by other factors, including previous experiences with health professionals and satisfaction with care, attitudes to self-medication, the use of alternative therapies and practitioners (Pill 1987; Telles and Pollack 1981), and worries about discovering the truth about symptoms relating to feared conditions such as cancer (Sheikh and Ogden 1998).

Qualitative studies are not based on formal models of help-seeking but often lead to an understanding of how different factors interact to determine whether services are accessed and the timing of professional-help-seeking. For example, detailed discussions with parents of the reasons for non-immunisation depict this as largely due to parents choosing not to immunise as a result of their assessment and balancing of the risks of side-effects, a belief in increased susceptibility to disease following immunisation, a belief in alternative protection such as homeopathic treatment, and practical reasons such as a lack of time (Sportan and Francis 2001). A qualitative study of barriers to the uptake of services for coronary heart disease for people with angina living in a deprived area of England identified six factors that prevented or delayed contact with professional services and referral to secondary care. These were: *service-related factors* (e.g. problems of access where transport was poor, inconvenient surgery times and perceptions of the GP as always busy), *personal factors* (fear and denial), *social and cultural factors* (e.g. the valuing of strength and an ability to cope, and maintaining independence), *past experiences and expectations* (e.g. previous problems accessing health care and bad experiences of health services), *diagnostic confusion* (problems associated with more prevailing and disabling health problems), and *lack of knowledge* and awareness of the causes, treatment and risks of heart disease (Tod *et al.* 2001). Similar broad groups of factors have been identified in other settings, although their content and importance varies for different populations and medical conditions. For example, a study to examine the low uptake of services by elderly people aged 75 years and over identified important factors contributing to non-uptake as: service-related (perceived service failure and costs), personal (embarrassment, fear of consequences), social and cultural (resignation, withdrawal and problem minimisation), past experiences and expectations (low expectations of services), and lack of knowledge/information of service availability (Walters *et al.* 2001).

Qualitative patient-centred studies have been important in demonstrating patients' and parents' own rationality and reasons for actions in terms of their beliefs, worries, expectations and uncertainties, and their perceptions of the costs and benefits of service use. This has been associated with and has encouraged a shift in emphasis from the goal of achieving greater patient conformity with professional definitions of appropriate service use to the increasing adoption of a patient-centred approach to service provision. This involves taking greater account of the public's and patients' perceived needs for professional advice and patterns of access to care in developing new forms of service provision, and ensuring that health promotion material addresses issues of concern for patients (see section on recent policies and service provision).

Social strategy approach

Pescosolido and colleagues have developed a framework termed the Social Organisation Strategy (SOS) for understanding people's health actions and use of services and regard this as responding to what they identify as limitations of previous approaches (Pescosolido 1992; Pescosolido and Kronenfeld 1995). They argue that although social networks have been acknowledged to influence professional-help-seeking, with a classic early study undertaken by Zola (1973), the embeddedness of problems and their solutions within the social network has been given insufficient attention. Following Freidson (1970) they regard the network interactions of individuals as driving the process of deciding whether something is wrong, whether anything can be done and what should be done, and how to evaluate the results. Pescosolido (1992) further criticises previous approaches to help-seeking for what she describes as the implicit emphasis on uncovering individuals' rational cost–benefit calculations as the engine of action. She argues that in reality social action often proceeds through cultural routines and habits, and may involve 'muddling through' and in some cases coercion (especially in relation to mental health services) rather than choice. Much social action is therefore outside the traditional rational-choice decision-making framework. Previous approaches (particularly quantitative models) are further viewed as overly static, focusing on one action at a time as a 'choice' or 'decision', and therefore ignoring how sequences of events are patterned, contingent and emergent. The recent emphasis on small-scale qualitative studies has to some extent overcome this and provided rich description. Pescosolido and colleagues however criticise this research for lacking explanation, and attribute this to the focus on individual agency which limits opportunities to uncover relevant social structural influences. Instead, Pescosolido and colleagues depict decision-making as a 'dynamic, interactive process that is fundamentally intertwined with the structured rhythms of social life' (Pescosolido et al. 1998: 1105). They regard the way forward as involving a synthesis of structural and process (social action) approaches in terms of the SOS. The SOS is described as an explicitly dynamic, network-centred, event-based approach that derives from four basic assumptions and building blocks:

1) the actor is seen as social and pragmatic rather than isolated and ever consciously rational; 2) the focus is shifted from the individual to the individual in patterned interaction with others; 3) the proper unit of analysis is the network, in recognition that the individual is embedded in an ongoing relational dynamic; 4) the context includes time and place, which represent different substantive and structural networks and form part of the embeddedness.

The focus of decision-making in the SOS, as with earlier stages' models, comprises the patterns, combinations or sequences of choices or decisions over the course of the episode, and how they are socially organised. However, in contrast with the depiction of decision-making as a linear sequence of events, largely removed from other aspects of daily life, the SOS regards this as a dynamic, iterative and multi-phased process that is 'masted on the back of ongoing social processes'. Health care decisions thus form one aspect of general decisions and demands of everyday life and its social interactions. This orientation towards process is accompanied by the need to know how lay, folk and professional resources assist in coping with a particular set of health problems over time, and in research terms requires the use of multilevel models (Pescosolido and Kronenfeld 1995).

The SOS framework has been tested using data from the 1975–6 US National Survey of Access to Health Care (Pescosolido 1992). Different care pathways among different groups in the population were identified using multinomial logit models to take account of the polytomous dependent variables (different courses of action). This identified the importance of varying sources of advice among different groups in the population. For example, black patients were found to be more likely to use physician-only strategies or to combine physicians and friends, and least likely to employ the strategy that combines physicians, the family and non-prescription drugs. Older people were more likely to use this latter strategy and were also most likely to rely only on a physician. In terms of the social network opportunity structure, people who were working were more likely to consult co-workers (in addition to the family and physician) or friends (in addition to the physician), and less likely to report that they do nothing about their condition. Married people were least likely to use strategies that incorporate friends or co-workers and relied more heavily on the family than other groups. Individuals with chronic or severe illness were more likely than other people to employ strategies with friends (in combination with physicians), family members (in combination with physicians), and the physician alone, and were least likely to rely on home remedies or the family alone. People with severe illnesses were also least likely to do nothing or employ strategies incorporating non-prescription drugs. As Pescosolido (1992) observed, this approach begins to identify the meaning and role of social life in help-seeking. It indicates that social characteristics (e.g. age, income, work status) may not distinguish those who consult from those who do not, but instead separates individuals who employ different strategies, which, sooner or later, involve consultation with a clinician. Pescosolido and colleagues (1998) further suggest that the notion of rational choice that traditionally underpinned utilisation studies is especially problematic in relation to mental health services. Using both a longitudinal data set and patients' 'stories' they identify the importance of three categories: 'choice' (individual and supported), coercion by family members or the police, and 'muddling through' with the lack of a clear agent. The importance of different strategies appeared to be influenced by the type of mental health problem and the characteristics of communities (Pescosolido *et al.* 1998).

Pescosolido's studies were undertaken in the US where most people have experienced a greater range of health choices, including the possibility of direct self-referral to a specialist service. However, Rogers and colleagues (1999) conducted a study informed by Pescosolido's framework in the north west region of the UK. This employed household interviews and four-week health diaries completed for 215 households. These data provided evidence of the influence of situational factors in containing illness, especially the demands of paid work. Only a small proportion of contacts with primary care were not preceded by attempts to ameliorate illness through self-care. Relatively few people were contacted for advice immediately prior to formal help-seeking but the authors point out that other people had a considerable influence over a longer time-scale. They describe lay knowledge about illness and health action as being gained over a long period and 'stored up' for use when needed.

Studies in the UK of doctors' behaviours when they themselves are ill also identified the role of both learned group norms, particularly the expectation that doctors would 'work through illness', as well as the immediate support and assistance provided by their network of medical colleagues at work (McKevitt and Morgan 1997a; 1997b). Doctors' illness behaviours were thus a product of their current and previous interactions with work colleagues, which as Pescosolido notes forms an important part of social networks for many people, as well as being influenced by the immediate organisational demands and difficulties of organising cover at short notice. Doctors also described a situation of managing and coping, conforming to Pescosolido's notion of 'muddling through', rather than making rational choices.

The SOS framework thus provides an important shift in emphasis. It both acknowledges health actions as often non-deliberative, undertaken in the context of the demands and circumstances of everyday life, and broadens the focus to include a diversity of informal and formal sources of advice and treatment that may be called on both prior to and following professional medical care rather than regarding self-treatment, the use of medical services and complementary medicines as separate areas of enquiry. Identification of the pathways that characterise different social groups and medical conditions requires to be complemented by detailed study of the circumstances, nature and content of health actions as an ongoing process.

Recent policies and service provision

The NHS policy framework traditionally aimed to encourage more appropriate patient behaviours within the prevailing framework and structure of service provision. This involved educational approaches to increase patients' medical knowledge, measures to achieve greater equity in provision, especially among socio-economically deprived populations (see Chapter 3), and measures to respond to specific barriers such as communication difficulties and a lack of efficient recall and reminders of preventive checks. A recent shift in NHS policies has involved the wider adoption of a patient-centred philosophy and approach to service provision, with the aim of building a health service that is ' responsive and sensitive to the needs of patients and the wider public' (Department of Health 1999). This involves greater public involvement in priority setting, patient-participation in decisions about treatment (shared decision-making), and ensuring that information and service provision take account of patients' own beliefs, priorities and behaviours. The aim is also to assist people in their choices and management of both medically trivial conditions and more serious disorders through providing more graduated access to services. This shift in emphasis can be illustrated by new approaches to A&E services. The traditional approach in the NHS was to define cases of 'inappropriate' attendance at A&E departments as a 'problem' to be discouraged through both informal and formal mechanisms, including providing educational leaflets about the appropriate use of services and refusing care to A&E attenders based on explicit assessment criteria. In contrast, recent initiatives have involved basing general practitioners within A&E departments in inner city areas to provide primary care services following triage undertaken by a nurse. This represents a shift from what Murphy (1998b) describes as '…vainly attempting to make the patients appropriate to the service' to concentrating on 'making the A&E service more appropriate to the patient' (p. 36). Patient-based approaches are also developing in other areas of health care. They include allowing patients to choose a suitable date and time for an outpatient appointment to suit their own circumstances with the aim of reducing problems of non-attendance (Sharp and Hamilton 2001), and developing graduated levels of primary care services to meet the varying needs of patients and support self-care, rather than general practitioners forming the sole entry point and source of provision (Coulter 1998). This has involved an expanded role for community pharmacists and the provision of advice and services by nurses in different primary settings. The latter include the setting up in 1998 of NHS Direct, which is a nurse-staffed national 24-hour telephone help-line to direct callers to the most appropriate service, advise on home care or give other advice (see Chapter 5). Other developments include the piloting of nurse-run clinics, the development of walk-in centres that can be used on a drop-in basis for minor treatment, and a proposed extension of the role of community pharmacists to support people in their illness management (Hassell *et al.* 1997). These approaches build on knowledge of patients' illness behaviours, including the substantial amount of self-care undertaken, and recognition that professional-help-seeking often represents a need for advice and support in situations of uncertainty. Small changes in patient behaviours through supporting self-management and providing graduated access to services are also regarded as having the potential to substantially reduce demands on medical staff and waiting times for those requiring these services (Rogers *et al.* 1998). Supporting self-management in turn requires increasing access to written information that is clearly presented, evidence-based and sufficiently comprehensive to allow people to take informed decisions, as well as providing advice through telephone help-lines, community pharmacists and other sources. Developments in patient information are therefore recognised as central to the new NHS strategy (Department of Health 1997, 1999).

The responsibility placed in the UK on health authorities and trusts to meet the needs of local populations has led to a number of new initiatives designed to increase access to services (Paterson and Judge 2002; Cooper *et al.* 2002). Many of these aim to reduce barriers to the use of mainstream services for disadvantaged groups through interventions such as reminder letters, telephone contact and health promotion campaigns to increase uptake of preventive services, and the provision of interpreter services and linkworkers. Another approach is to provide special services for groups who have particular difficulties in using formal services, such as outreach care in hostels and day centres for homeless people. Local initiatives in reducing barriers to care are complemented by national strategies such as flexible contractual arrangements by which GPs and allied staff deliver personal medical services to underserved groups, including elderly, mentally ill and homeless people, and those in deprived or low-income areas (Lewis *et al.* 1999).

This section has focused specifically on NHS policies but similar trends are evident in many health systems. This includes an increasing emphasis on a patient-centred framework and ensuring that services are accessible and acceptable to local populations (Paterson and Judge 2002).

Conclusions

Patients' help-seeking behaviours have been shown to play a key role in determining when and how services are accessed. Neither the presence of signs and symptoms nor the simple availability of services are in themselves sufficient to explain whether and when service use occurs and even where, as in the NHS, medical care is free at the point of use, only a minority of people visit the doctor without first undertaking other health actions. A number of explanatory frameworks and approaches have been developed to explain patient behaviours and draw attention to different aspects of a complex social reality. Some focus on individual decision-making and emphasise the influence of beliefs, expectations, worries and uncertainties in managing symptoms and professional-help-seeking. Other approaches emphasise structural barriers relating to financial aspects, the organisation and provision of health care and general cultural beliefs and attitudes to health and health care. The social organisation strategy aims to bring together structure and social action with its emphasis on the embeddedness of health problems and actions in the context of the demands of everyday life and social networks. These frameworks have general applicability, although the importance of particular beliefs and barriers depends on systems of financing and service provision and the wider social and cultural context of health care.

A particular focus of studies of help-seeking behaviours has been to explain differences in the uptake and timing of service use among social groups defined in terms of socio-economic status, age, ethnicity and gender, as well as the special situation of institutional populations. This has drawn attention to the range of barriers and circumstances that impact on help-seeking by disadvantaged groups, and the differences between local areas in the composition, circumstances and needs of their populations. It has led to a recognition that the provision of services will not in itself achieve equity of uptake and outcomes unless responsive to the specific concerns and barriers experienced by different groups of potential patients, and considerable emphasis is given to identifying and responding to local needs as well as to broader policies to increase the accessibility and quality of services.

For the future, patients' uptake of services is likely to take place in an increasingly differentiated health system in terms of sources and sites of professional care. This raises questions about the pathways to care of different patient groups, in the context of the increased availability of telephone advice and the greater availability of nurse-led services and alternative treatments. Developments in possibilities of remote access to specialist services through telemedicine will also present both new barriers and opportunities and may have a differential impact on social groups. It is therefore important that future assessments of access pay greater attention to patients' differing points of entry and their journeys through the health system, with initial entry not necessarily guaranteeing access to expensive technologies and specialised services.

References

Ajzen, I. and Fishbein, M. (1970) 'The prediction of behaviour from attitudinal and normative beliefs', *J Pers Soc Psychol*, 6: 466–87.

Andersen, R.M. (1968) *Behavioural Model of Families' Use of Health Services*, Research Series No. 25. Chicago, IL: Centre for Health Administration Studies, University of Chicago.

Andersen, R.M. (1995) 'Revisiting the behavioural model and access to care: does it matter?', *Journal of Health and Social Behaviour*, 36: 1–10.

Andersen, R.M. and Newman, J. (1973) 'Societal and individual determinants of medical care utilization', *Milbank Memorial Fund Quarterly*, 51: 95–124.

Arber, S., Gilbert, N. and Dale, A. (1985) 'Paid employment and women's health: a benefit or a source of role strain?', *Sociology of Health and Illness*, 7: 375–99.

Atkinson, M., Clark, M., Clay, D., Johnson, M., Owen, D. and Szczepura, A. (2001) *Systematic Review of Ethnicity and Health Service Access for London*. Warwick: Centre for Health services Research (University of Warwick), Mary Seacole Research Centre (de Montfort University), Centre for Research in Ethnic Relations (University of Warwick).

Barbour, R. (1999) 'The case for combining qualitative and quantitative approaches in health services research', *Journal of Health Services Research and Policy*, 14: 39–43.

Becker, M.H. and Maiman, L.A. (1975) 'Socio-behavioural determinants of compliance with health and medical care recommendations', *Medical Care*, 13: 10–24.

Becker, M.H., Haefner, D.P., Kasl, S.V., Kirscht, J., Maiman, L. and Rosenstock, I.M. (1977) 'Selected psychological models and correlates of individual health related behaviours', *Medical Care*, 15(5) supplement: 27–46.

Birkhead, J.S. (1992) 'Time delays in the provision of thrombolytic treatment in six district hospitals, Joint Audit Committee of the British Cardiac Society and Cardiology Committee of the Royal College of Physicians of London', *British Medical Journal*, 305: 445–8.

Calnan, M. (1982) 'The hospital accident and emergency department: what is its role?', *Journal of Social Policy*, 2: 483–503.

Calnan, M. (1984) 'The health belief model and participation in programmes for the early detection of breast cancer: a comparative analysis', *Social Science and Medicine*, 19: 823–30.

Calnan, M. and Johnson, B. (1985) 'Health, health risks and inequalities: an exploratory study of women's perceptions', *Sociology of Health and Illness*, 7(1): 55–75.

Campbell, J.L. (1994) 'General practitioner appointment systems, patient satisfaction, and the use of accident and emergency services: a study in one geographical area', *Family Practice*, 11: 438–45.

Campbell, J.L. and Roland, M.O. (1996) 'Why do people consult the doctor?', *Family Practice*, 13: 75–83.

Carlisle, R., Groom, L., Avery, A., Boot, D. and Earwicker, S. (1998) 'Relation of out of hours activity by general practice and accident and emergency services with deprivation in Nottingham: longitudinal survey', *British Medical Journal*, 316: 520–3.

Conner, M. and Norman, P. (1996) *Predicting Health Behaviour*. Buckingham: Open University Press.

Cooper, L.A., Hill, M.N. and Powe N.R. (2002) 'Designing and evaluating interventions to eliminate racial and ethnic disparities in health care', *Journal of General Internal Medicine*, 17: 477–86.

Coulter, A. (1998) 'Managing demand at the interface between primary and secondary care', *British Medical Journal*, 316: 174–6.

Crane, M. and Warnes, A.M. (2001) 'Primary health care services for single homeless people: defects and opportunities', *Family Practice*, 18(3): 272–6.

Davison, C., Davey Smith, G., Frankel, S. (1991) 'Lay epidemiology and the prevention paradox: the implications of coronary candidacy for health education', *Sociology of Health and Illness*, 13(1): 1–19.

Delaney, B.C. (1998) 'Why do dyspeptic patients over the age of 50 consult their general practitioner? A qualitative investigation of health beliefs relating to dyspepsia', *British Journal of General Practice*, 433: 1481–5.

Department of Health (1997) *The New NHS: Modern, Dependable*. London: HMSO.

Department of Health (1999) *Cervical Screening Programme, England: 1998–99*. London: Department of Health. Bulletin 1999/32.2000.

Department of Health (2000) *Breast Screening Programme, England:1998–99*. London: Department of Health. Bulletin 2000/7.2000.

Doyal, L. (1994) 'Waged work and well-being'. In S. Wilkinson and S. Kitzinger (eds) *Women and Health*, pp.65–84. London: Taylor and Francis.

Feder, G., Crook, A.M., Magee, P., Banerjee, S., Timmis, A.D. and Hemingway, H. (2002) 'Ethnic differences in invasive management of coronary disease: prospective cohort study of patients undergoing angiography', *British Medical Journal*, 324: 511–16.

Fergusson, E., Li, J. and Taylor, B. (1998) 'Grandmothers' role in preventing unnecessary accident and emergency attendances: cohort study', *British Medical Journal*, 317: 1685.

Fraser, S., Bunce, C., Wormaid, R. and Brunner, E. (2001) 'Deprivation and late presentation of glaucoma: case control study', *British Medical Journal*, 322: 639–43.

Free, C., White, P., Shipman, C. and Dale, J. (1999) 'Access to and use of out-of-hours services by members of Vietnamese community groups in South London: a focus group study', *Family Practice*, 16(4): 369–74.

Freidson, E. (1970) *The Profession of Medicine*. New York: Dodds Mead and Co.

Gillam, S.J. (1991) 'Understanding the uptake of cervical screening – the contribution of the health belief model', *British Journal of General Practice*, 41: 510–13.

Goddard, M. and Smith, P. (2001) 'Equity of access to health services: theory and evidence from the UK', *Social Science and Medicine*, 53: 1149–62.

Green, J. and Dale, J. (1992) 'Primary care in accident and emergency and general practice: a comparison', *Social Science and Medicine*, 35(8): 987–1005.

Hallam, L. (1994) 'Primary health care outside normal working hours: review of published work', *British Medical Journal*, 308: 249–53.

Hannay, D.R. (1979) *The Symptom Iceberg: A Study of Community Health*. London: Routledge and Kegan Paul.

Harrison, J.A., Mullen, P.D. and Green, L.W. (1992) 'A meta-analysis of studies of the health belief model with adults', *Health Education Research, Theory and Practice*, 7: 107–16.

Hassell, K., Noyce, P., Rogers, A., Harris, J. and Wilkinson, J. (1997) 'A pathway to the GP: the pharmaceutical "consultation" as the first port of call in primary health care', *Family Practice*, 14: 498–502.

Haynes, R. (1991) 'Inequalities in health and health service use from the General Household Survey', *Social Science and Medicine*, 33: 361–8.

Heywood, P.L., Blackie, G.C., Cameron, I.H. and Dowell, A.C. (1998) 'An assessment of the attributes of frequent attenders to general practice', *Family Practice*, 15(3): 198–204.

Janz, N. and Becker, M.H. (1984) 'The health belief model: a decade later', *Health Education Quarterly*, 11: 1–47.

Jiwa, M. (2000) 'Frequent attenders in general practice: an attempt to reduce attendance', *Family Practice*, 17: 248–51.

Joint Prison Service and NHS Executive Working Group (1999) *The Future Organisation of Prison Health Care*. London: HM Prison Service and NHS Executive.

Jones, D. and Gill, P.S. (1998) 'Refugees and primary care: tackling the inequalities', *British Medical Journal*, 317: 1444–6.

Jones, J. (1999) 'Breast cancer treatment delays affect survival', *British Medical Journal*, 318: 919.

Kai, J. (1996) 'Parents' difficulties and information needs in coping with acute illness in pre-school children: a qualitative study', *British Medical Journal*, 313: 987–90.

Kavanagh, S. and Knapp, M. (1998) 'The impact on general practitioners of the changing balance of care for elderly people living in institutions', *British Medical Journal*, 317: 322–7.

Kavanagh, S. and Knapp, M. (1999) 'Primary care arrangements for elderly people in residential and nursing homes (letter)', *British Medical Journal*, 318: 666.

Killaspy, H., Banerjee, S., King, M. and Lloyd, M. (1999) 'Non-attendance at psychiatric outpatient clinics: communication and implications for primary care', *British Journal of General Practice*, 49: 880–3.

Kookier, S. (1995) 'Exploring the iceberg of morbidity: a comparison of different survey methods for assessing the occurrence of everyday illness', *Social Science and Medicine*, 17(3): 147–61.

Koos, E.L. (1954). *The Health of Regionville*. New York: Columbia University Press.

Last, J.M. (1963) 'The iceberg: completing the clinical picture in general practice', *Lancet*, ii: 28–31.

Leslie, W.S., Urie, A., Hooper, J. and Morrisson, C.E. (2000) 'Delay in calling for help during myocardial infarction: reasons for delay and subsequent patterns of accessing care', *Heart*, 84: 137–41.

Lewis, R., Jenkins, C. and Gillam, S. (1999) *Personal Medical Services Pilots in London: Rewriting the Red Book*. London: The King's Fund.

Lynch, M. (1995) 'Effect of practice and patient population characteristics on the uptake of childhood immunisations', *British Journal of General Practice*, 45: 205–8.

McKevitt, C. and Morgan, M. (1997a) 'Sickness absence and working through illness: a comparison of two professional groups', *Journal of Public Health Medicine*, (3): 295–300.

McKevitt, C. and Morgan, M. (1997b) 'Illness doesn't belong to us', *Journal of Royal Society of Medicine*, 90: 491–5.

Mechanic, D. (1962) 'The concept of illness behaviour', *Journal of Chronic Diseases*, 15: 189–94.

Meyer-Weitz, A., Reddy, P., Van den Borne, H.W., Kok, G. and Pietersen J. (2000) 'Health care seeking behaviour with sexually transmitted diseases: determinants of delay behaviour', *Patient Education and Counselling*, 41: 263–74.

Morgan, M. (2003) 'The doctor–patient relationship'. In G. Scambler (ed) *Sociology as Applied to Medicine*. London: W.B. Saunders.

Morris, C.J., Cantrill, J.A. and Weiss, M.C. (2001) 'GPs' attitudes to minor ailments', *Family Practice*, 18(6): 581–5.

Murphy, A.W. (1998a) '"Inappropriate" attenders at accident and emergency departments I: Definition, incidence and reasons for attendance', *Family Practice*, 15(1): 23–32.

Murphy, A.W. (1998b) '"Inappropriate" attenders at accident and emergency departments II: Health service responses. *Family Practice* 15(1): 33–7.

Naish, J. (1994) 'Intercultural consultations: investigating factors that deter non-English speaking women from attending their general practitioners for cervical screening', *British Medical Journal*, 309: 1126–29.

National Audit Office (1992) *NHS Accident and Emergency Departments in England*. London: HMSO.

Neal, R.D., Lawlor, D., Allgar, V., College, M., Shahid, A., Hassey, A., Portz, C. and Wilson, A. (2001) 'Missed appointments in general practice: retrospective data analysis from four practices', *British Journal of General Practice*, 51: 830–2.

Nemet, G.F. and Bailey, A.J. (2000) 'Distance and health care utilization among the rural elderly', *Social Science and Medicine*, 50: 1197–208.

Nguyen-Van-Tam, J.S. and Baker, D.M. (1992) 'General practice and accident and emergency department care: does the patient know best?', *British Medical Journal*, 305: 157–8.

Paterson, I. and Judge, K. (2002) 'Equality of access to health care'. In J.P. Mackenbach and M.J. Bakker (eds) *Socio-economic Inequalities in Health in Europe*. London: Routledge.

Payne, N. and Saul, C. (1997) 'Variations in use of cardiology services in a health authority: comparison of coronary artery revascularisation rates with prevalence of angina and coronary mortality', *British Medical Journal*, 314: 257.

Pescosolido, B.A. (1992) 'Beyond rational choice: the social dynamics of how people seek help', *American Journal of Sociology*, 97(4): 1096–138.

Pescosolido, B.A., Gardner, B. and Lubell, K. (1998) 'How people get into mental health services: stories of choice, coercion and "muddling through" from first timers', *Social Science and Medicine*, 46(2): 275–86.

Pescosolido, B.A. and Kronenfeld, J.J. (1995) 'Health, illness, and healing in an uncertain era: challenges from and for medical sociology', *Journal of Health and Social Behaviour*, 35: 5–33.

Pill, R. (1987) 'Models and management: the case of cystitis in women', *Sociology of Health and Illness*, 9(3): 265–86.

Plearce, N. and Quilgares, D. (1996) *Health and Homelessness in London*. London: King's Fund.

Power, R., French, R. and Connelly, J. (1999) 'Health, health promotion and homelessness', *British Medical Journal*, 318: 590–2.

Prince, M. and Worth, C. (1992) 'A study of "inappropriate" attendances to a paediatric accident and emergency department', *Journal of Public Health Medicine*, 14: 177–82.

Public Health Laboratory Service Communicable Disease Surveillance Centre (2001) *Communicable Disease Report Weekly*, 11(39): immunisation; available http://www.phls.org.uk/publications/CDR%20Weekly/PDF%20files/2001/cdr3901.pdf.

Reading, R., Colver, A., Openshaw, S. and Jarvis, S. (1994) 'Do interventions that improve immunisation uptake also reduce social inequalities in uptake?', *British Medical Journal*, 308: 1142–4.

Reed, J.L. and Lyne, M. (1997) 'The quality of health care in prison: results of a years programme of semi-structured inspections', *British Medical Journal*, 315: 1420–4.

Reed, J.L. and Lyne, M. (2000) 'Inpatient care of mentally ill people in prison: results of a year's programme of semi-structured inspections', *British Medical Journal*, 318: 954–5.

Richards, H., Reid, M.E. and Watts, G.C.M. (2002) 'Socio-economic variations in responses to chest pain: qualitative study', *British Medical Journal*, 324: 1308–11

Roberts, H. (1992) 'Professionals' and parents' perceptions of A-and-E use in a children's hospital', *Sociological Review*, 40(1): 109–31.

Robertson-Steel, I.R.S. (1998) 'Providing primary care in the accident and emergency department (editorial)', *British Medical Journal*, 316: 409–10.

Robinson, J.K., Altman, J.S. and Rademaker, A.W. (1995) 'Socioeconomic status and attitudes of 51 patients with giant basal and squamous cell carcinoma and paired controls', *Archives of Dermatology*, 131: 428–43.

Rogers, A., Entwistle,V. and Pencheon, D. (1998) 'A patient-led NHS: managing demand at the interface between lay and primary care', *British Medical Journal*, 316: 1816–19.

Rogers, A., Hassell, K. and Nicholas, G. (1999) *Demanding Patients? Analysing the Use of Primary Care*. Buckingham: Open University.

Rogers, R.W. (1975) 'A protection motivation theory of appeals and attitude change', *Journal of Psychology*, 91: 93–114.

Rosenstock, I. (1966) 'Why people use health services', *Milbank Memorial Fund Quarterly*, 44: 94–127.

Rosenstock, I. (1974) 'The health belief model and preventive health behaviour', *Health Education Monographs*, 2: 354–86.

Ruston, A., Clayton, J. and Calnan, M. (2000) 'Patients' action during their cardiac event: qualitative study exploring differences and modifiable factors', *British Medical Journal*, 316: 1060–5.

Sharp, D.J. and Hamilton, W. (eds) (2001) 'Non-attendance at general practices and outpatient clinics', *British Medical Journal*, 323: 1081–2.

Shaw, C.M., Creed, F., Tomenson, B., Riste, L. and Cruickshank, J.K. (1999) 'Prevalence and anxiety and depressive illness and help-seeking behaviour in African Caribbeans and white Europeans: two phase general population survey', *British Medical Journal*, 318: 302–6.

Shaw, C., Tansey, R., Jackson, C., Hyde, C. and Allan, R. (2001) 'Barriers to help-seeking in people with urinary symptoms', *Family Practice*, 18: 48–52.

Sheikh, I. and Ogden, J. (1998) 'The role of knowledge and beliefs in help seeking behaviour for cancer: a quantitative and qualitative approach', *Patient Education and Counselling*, 35: 35–42.

Shipman, C., Payne, F., Dale, J. and Jessop, L. (2001) 'Patient-perceived benefits of and barriers to using out-of-hours primary care centres', *Family Practice*, 18(2): 149–55.

Smith, R. (ed) (1999) 'Medicine and the marginalized (editorial)', *British Medical Journal*, 319: 1589–90.

Sporton, R.K. and Francis, S.A. (2001) 'Choosing not to immunize: are parents making informed decisions?', *Family Practice*, 18(2): 181–8.

Steinmetz, D. and Tabenkin, H. (2001) 'The "difficult" patient as perceived by family physicians', *Family Practice*, 18(5): 495–500.

Telles, B. and Pollack, M. (1981) 'Feeling sick: the experience and legitimation of illness', *Social Science and Medicine,* 15(9): 243–51.

Tod, A.M., Read, C., Lacey, A. and Abbott, J. (2001) 'Barriers to uptake of services for coronary heart disease: qualitative study', *British Medical Journal*, 323: 214–17.

Tudor Hart, J. (1971) 'The inverse care law', *Lancet*, I, 405–12.

Van de Lisdonk, E.H. (1989) 'Perceived and presented morbidity in general practice', *Scandinavian Journal of Primary Health Care*, 7: 73–8.

Van der Kar A., Knottnerus, A., Meertens, R., Dubois V. and Kok, G. (1992) 'Why do patients consult the general practitioner? Determinants of their decision', *British Journal of General Practice*, 42: 313–16.

Wadsworth, M., Butterfield, W. and Blaney, R. (1971) *Health and Sickness: The Choice of Treatment*. London: Tavistock.

Walsh, M. (1995) 'The health belief model and use of accident and emergency services by the general public', *Journal of Advanced Nursing*, 22(4): 694–9.

Walters, K., Iliffe, S. and Orrell, M. (2001) 'An exploration of help-seeking behaviour in older people with unmet needs', *Family Practice*, 18(3): 277–82.

Wells, B.L. and Horm, J.W.(1992) 'Stages at diagnosis in breast cancer: race and socio-economic factors', *American Journal of Public Health*, 82: 1383–5.

Yabroff, K.R. and Mandelblatt, J.S. (1999) 'Interventions targeted towards patients to increase mammography use', *Cancer Epidemiology Biomarkers and Prevention*, 8: 749–57.

Zola, I.K. (1973) 'Pathways to the doctor: from person to patient', *Social Science and Medicine*, 7: 677–89.

Chapter 5

Organisational barriers to access

Roger Beech

Introduction

If the use of health services is to result in satisfactory health outcomes, appropriate, timely and effective health care is required. A particular concern in the UK is that people may not be able to gain access to the services that they need in a timely manner. In a survey of over 150,000 people, waiting for NHS care was identified as the public's most important concern in relation to access. Problems included waiting to see primary care staff, waiting for hospital appointments, waiting in hospital accident and emergency departments, waiting to be admitted to hospital, and waiting to be discharged from hospital (Department of Health 2000a).

From a health system perspective, a major determinant of long waiting times for health care in a centrally funded service is the overall level of funding of health care and thus the availability of hospital beds, medical and nursing staff or pharmaceutical budgets. Spending on health care in the NHS as a proportion of gross domestic product, is lower in the UK than in many other comparable countries. Waiting lists have traditionally been viewed as one of the mechanisms used to ration the delivery of care in a system which is free at the point of use (Foster 1983). However, there is also an increasing appreciation of the importance of organisational deficiencies in the ways that existing capacity and resources are delivered and managed that accentuate the impacts of an overall shortfall in capacity. This has led to a growing interest in 'redesigning' services so as to improve patient access.

This chapter addresses both initial access, and access to different levels of care, across different services. It provides evidence of organisational barriers to access, especially in terms of long waiting lists and times for NHS treatment. This focuses attention on ways of achieving greater efficiency and thus increasing service availability and reducing delays and other barriers in achieving access. The chapter then examines the cause of these problems, focusing particularly on organisational inefficiencies in the supply of health services. It also outlines the service developments that are being introduced in the NHS to address these problems and considers their likely impacts. The setting for this chapter is the NHS of the UK but comparative studies have shown that similar problems exist elsewhere, although waiting lists and delays in treatment may be less pronounced. A recent comparison of the NHS with an integrated system for financing and delivering health services (Kaiser Permanente) in California suggested that there were important differences in the organisation and delivery of services. For example, Kaiser members received more comprehensive and convenient primary care services and much more rapid access to specialist services and hospital admissions (Feacham *et al.* 2002). A key question concerns the differences in costs of the two systems, but the interpretation of cost estimates in this study was controversial.

Problems of service delivery

Organisational problems represent a fairly universal characteristic of health systems but the ones identified as being important vary over time and between countries. Organisational problems include a lack of investment and resources in terms of beds, staff, theatre availability or other aspects of service provision required to meet patients' needs. Poor management frequently compounds the problems of service availability. This may involve a lack of appropriate application of technology, poor co-ordination between staff groups and sectors, and the power of doctors and other groups within the system to promote their sectional interests.

Primary care

The main concerns with access in primary care include the ability to register with a general practitioner of choice, the ability to obtain a timely appointment, and the ability to access care outside working hours. A survey of 1,139 adults in London organised by the King's Fund found that 86 per cent of respondents found it easy to register with their current GP, and 70 per cent said they had registered with their first choice of doctor (Malbon *et al.* 2000). Groups who have particular difficulty registering with a GP include homeless people, drug users and others who are considered to be demanding or anti-social (see Chapter 4). A survey of a random sample of general practitioners in England and Wales also indicated that 40 per cent had removed one or more patients in the previous six months, with the main reasons stated as threatening or abusive behaviour, a complaint by a patient, and failure to take up preventive services that are subject to GP performance targets (Pickin *et al.* 2001).

Difficulty in obtaining an appointment to see a GP is also an important concern. The King's Fund survey showed that around 50 per cent of respondents were unhappy with the time that it took them to get an appointment to consult a GP during normal working hours; 79 per cent said that they would not be able to get a non-urgent appointment on the same day, 82 per cent that they would not obtain an appointment within two days, and around 28 per cent said that they would have to wait more than three days (Malbon *et al.* 2000). Having to wait more than three days is widespread, with appointment schedules often being saturated for a week or more in advance. This causes difficulties for patients and practice staff (particularly receptionists) and capacity may be used inefficiently because many patients do not attend for their booked consultation and may have improved or obtained care elsewhere before their appointment.

The level of demand for out-of-hours care from general practices is substantial. There has been a trend to meet this by GPs using deputising services or grouping together into co-operatives to provide out-of-hours care. However, patients appear to be less satisfied by care provided by a deputising service compared with their own GP (McKinley et al. 1997).

Emergency acute care

There is currently an upward trend in emergency admissions to acute care, especially amongst those over 65 years of age. Between 1989 and 1994, the number of emergency admissions per head of population increased by 2.1 per cent (and by 3.3 per cent for those over 65) and from 1994 to 1998 by 2 per cent (and by 2.7 per cent for those over 65). All overnight admissions (elective and emergency cases combined) have also risen: by 1.6 per cent per annum from 1980 to 1994 and by 1.9 per cent per annum from 1994 to 1998 (Department of Health 2000b).

In spite of these increases in demand, the 1980s and 1990s also saw a downward trend in hospital bed numbers. The number of general and acute hospital beds available fell by 2.6 per cent per annum from 1980 to 1994, and by 1.9 per cent per annum from 1994 to 1998 (Department of Health 2000b). Higher acute hospital bed occupancy rates and reductions in average lengths of stay both helped to offset the effects of the rise in demand. There has also been a substantial increase in procedures conducted on a day case rather than inpatient basis as a result of less invasive techniques.

Towards the end of the 1990s, problems began to emerge. The downward trend in lengths of stay flattened and possibly reversed (NHS Executive West Midlands 1998). In addition, hospital occupancy rates of around 90 per cent (Department of Health 2001a) were not sustainable and created instability within the system of services for providing emergency care. When average occupancy rates exceed 85 per cent there is a rapid increase in the difficulties that hospitals face in responding to the peaks and troughs of demands for acute care (Bagust et al. 1999; NHS Executive 1998). As a result many hospitals found that they had insufficient beds to admit those patients who needed emergency care. Difficulties in obtaining access to beds for specialist intensive care were also reported (NHS Executive 1998; Scrivens et al. 1999). The shortage of beds for admissions also created problems in hospital accident and emergency departments: patients had to be accommodated on trolleys while they waited for a hospital bed to become available. During November and December 1999, 2,361 individuals had to spend more than 12 hours on a trolley waiting to be admitted, and 108 individuals over 24 hours (corresponding figures for November and December 2001 are 806 and zero) (Department of Health 2002). There were also knock-on effects in terms of long waiting times in accident and emergency departments for those individuals who did not require admission. It is hardly surprising then that when surveyed as part of the development of the NHS Plan, 60 per cent of respondents thought that waits in accident and emergency departments were too long and that trolley waits were unacceptable (Department of Health 2000a).

In spite of these difficulties in gaining access to acute beds, it is common for a proportion of acute beds to be 'blocked' by patients who are waiting to be discharged from acute care: so called 'bed blockers'. The NHS Plan included a survey of 5,500 over-75-year-olds who were waiting to be discharged from acute inpatient care, and identified considerable problems of access both within the system and between health and social services. Altogether 42 per cent of respondents were waiting to be discharged to a residential home. A further 23 per cent were waiting for an assessment of their on-going care needs prior to discharge and 6 per cent for a package of home care to be provided (Department of Health 2000a). Amongst elderly patients, McDonagh and colleagues concluded that around 20 per cent of acute bed use was probably avoidable, with moderate nursing care or long-term care being the preferred alternative (McDonagh *et al.* 2000).

Such findings indicate that difficulties in accessing acute beds for emergency care are being accentuated by poor co-ordination between the NHS and other agencies and the failure to care for some patients in alternative settings. Unfortunately, there is currently insufficient capacity to care for all such patients in alternative settings and, as a result, the national inquiry of acute bed use within the NHS concluded that,

> Current inpatient services do not match patients' needs as well as they should … The Inquiry has found evidence of significant inappropriate or avoidable use of acute hospital beds and of shortages of service alternatives to acute hospital care that could reduce admissions and bring care closer to or into patients' homes.
>
> (Department of Health 2000b: 6)

This problem of patients with non-acute needs occupying acute beds is also common elsewhere in Europe. Lorenzo and Sunol (1995) reviewed the findings of studies of acute bed use in Spain during the 1980s and 1990s. Reported levels of avoidable acute admissions ranged from 2.1 per cent to 44.8 per cent of admissions, whilst levels of avoidable days of care ranged from 15.0 per cent to 43.9 per cent of acute bed days. Delays in transferring patients to settings for follow-on care, and 'conservative' management by physicians, were seen as the main causes of avoidable acute bed use. Similar findings were reported by Fellin *et al.* (1995) in an overview of studies of acute bed use in Italy. Rates of avoidable acute admission ranged from 25 per cent to 38 per cent and of avoidable acute days of care from 28 per cent to 49 per cent. The main causes of avoidable acute bed use were delays in access to tests, investigations, and operating theatre facilities, and delays in transfer to long-term care.

Elective hospital care

The elective care system covers referral for assessment by a clinician at an outpatient clinic and, if required, subsequent referral for treatment as an outpatient, day case, or inpatient. Each type of referral involves patients being added to a 'waiting list' which highlights issues of access and barriers to care within the system once initial service contact has been made. Patients first wait for outpatient appointments and investigations and then, where necessary, wait for an inpatient procedure to be undertaken. It is these waits that have traditionally been a cause for concern within the NHS. Currently around 24 per cent of individuals referred for an outpatient appointment have to wait longer than three months to be seen. As of October 2001, out of an overall NHS inpatient waiting list of around one million individuals, 39,700 (4 per cent) had waited over 12 months for their elective procedure and 8,100 (0.9 per cent) over 15 months. (Wanless 2002; Department of Health 2002). Four specialties account for most of the long waits: orthopaedics, dermatology, ear, nose and throat problems, and eye conditions (Department of Health 2000a).

In the consumer survey conducted for the NHS Plan, 70 per cent of respondents thought that waiting lists and waiting times were too long (Department of Health 2000a). The Wanless report also includes findings which demonstrate that levels of public satisfaction with waiting fall sharply as waiting times increase. In a survey of public attitudes to outpatient waiting times, 50 per cent of individuals were satisfied with waits of up to two weeks, falling to 37 per cent for waits of up to three months, 10 per cent for up to six months, and 0 per cent for over six months (Wanless 2002). Long waiting times are also a major reason for the considerable increase in elective surgical procedures undertaken and paid for privately in the UK (or funded through private insurance schemes) (see Chapter 6).

Whilst lack of capacity for elective care is one reason for organisational barriers to access, organisational inefficiencies surrounding the management of existing capacity have also been highlighted. These include delays in the scheduling of tests and investigations, and poor scheduling of outpatient clinics, with patients being given similar appointment times. This practice reduces the likelihood of doctors having to wait for patients to arrive, but it immediately builds in a systematic delay for patients (Worthington 1997). Published research also indicates that many repeat visits for outpatient care may be avoidable (McKee et al. 2000; Teale et al. 2000; Frankel and Faulkner 1994), an effect that will lead to unnecessary increases in the lengths of waiting lists. There are also inefficiencies in the management of waiting lists, with the selection of types of cases from waiting lists often reflecting consultants' own particular interests and preferences rather than being determined by the composition of lists and clinical need. Admissions clerks may then select those patients more recently put on a waiting list as being more likely to still require the operation and not have moved, died or had the procedure privately, with the result that the waiting list becomes more like a pool than an orderly queue (Pope 1991).

In terms of the supply of services there is evidence of poor management of operating theatre sessions leading to a substantial under-use of capacity and a failure to reach targets of using 90 per cent of allocated theatre time. Common weaknesses are identified as poor management information systems, failure to restructure historic patterns of allocating operating theatre time, and consultants taking annual leave at short notice (Audit Commission 2002). Finally, poor planning of hospital capacity for emergency admissions can mean that beds for elective care have to be 'borrowed' by emergency admissions and as a result elective admissions and operations have to be cancelled (Department of Health 2001b; Department of Health 2001a).

Organisational responses

The NHS is a cash-limited system that has traditionally received a relatively small percentage of gross domestic product in terms of a European or broader international context (see Chapter 6). A continuing concern of the NHS has therefore been to meet demands by increased efficiency and thus achieve higher levels of service delivery within existing budgets. This has resulted in several reorganisations of the service while remaining a relatively centralised, tax-funded service, pledged to providing a comprehensive range of health services that is equally accessible to the whole population on the basis of need and largely free at the point of use. In particular the managerial reforms of 1983 gave priority to achieving greater efficiency and 'value for money' through increasing individual responsibility and accountability (Department of Health and Social Security 1983). A key aspect of this was the strengthening of management through establishing a hierarchy of general managers on fixed term contracts and paid according to their performance. These full-time managers began to introduce more controls over the way traditionally autonomous clinicians used the resources available to them. For example, clinicians became increasingly responsible and accountable for delivering an agreed workload efficiently within a set budget through systems of resource management. A system of quantitative performance indicators was also established to measure and compare the activity and costs of each district and hospital. A limited list of drugs of proven effectiveness which GPs were allowed to prescribe on the NHS was established, and a system of competitive tendering was introduced for support services, such as catering, cleaning and security (Packwood et al. 1991).

Following the 1983 reforms, the NHS continued to face the familiar problem of reconciling available funds with increasing demands generated by an ageing population and new technology. Resulting cash shortages forced some districts to close wards and cancel non-emergency admissions in order to stay within budget. Waiting lists, which had always been a cause of public concern, shot into the headlines (Mays 1997). A review of the NHS undertaken in 1988/9 identified a major organisational problem as the lack of incentives within the NHS for health care providers to be efficient, with the result that resources were not being used as well as they could be. For example, there was no incentive for hard-working staff in a hospital to become more productive and treat more patients, since the hospital budget would remain the same (see Chapter 6).

Major features of the NHS reforms implemented in 1991 were the creation of a purchaser–provider split ('internal market'), and the introduction of greater professional accountability, including compulsory, professionally-led audit of medical practice to ensure quality and efficient use of hospital resources and a strengthening of the system for monitoring GP prescribing and quality of care (Secretaries of State 1989). Under the internal market, health authorities became primarily purchasers not providers, buying hospital and community health services for their populations from providers in public, private or voluntary sectors. Hospitals were encouraged to apply for 'trust' status in which they remain in the NHS but have greater freedom to set up their own management arrangements. Trusts' income was based on their ability to market their services to purchasers (health authorities, GP fund-holders and private insurers), thus introducing an element of competition among providers in achieving contracts with implications for costs and quality. General practices were encouraged to become GP fund-holders and to take control of their own budgets for the non-emergency hospital care of the patients on their lists. The idea was that fund-holding practices would be more likely to challenge providers to produce better services than staff in health authorities and that 'unnecessary' hospital referrals would be reduced because they had placed a cost on the budgets of GP fund-holders.

The 1991 reforms increased administrative costs but also had some benefits. Providers became more aware of issues of cost and quality in their services, and purchasers were encouraged to contract for new forms of services more relevant to the needs of patients. These included the development of specialist outreach services in the community, the use of skilled nurse practitioners and shared care between the hospital and community (Mays 1997). However, as this chapter has shown, problems of waiting times and inefficiencies in the system remain and there are concerns about substantial variations in standards and waiting times in different parts of the country.

The current philosophy and approach to the NHS is outlined in the White Paper, *The New NHS: Modern Dependable* (Department of Health 1997) and the NHS Plan (Department of Health 2000a). These emphasise the creation of a system based on partnership by breaking down organisational barriers both within the NHS and between the NHS and other sectors, which is tailored to patients' needs and circumstances, and driven by performance with incentives and sanctions at all levels to improve efficiency. Fundamental changes include replacing the market mechanism with long-term service agreements, and giving increased emphasis to national quality standards including national standards for treating all major conditions. The problem of access to care will mainly be addressed in three ways: 1) increased investment in the NHS; 2) new ways of organising existing services, including new booking systems and targets for waiting times, and national standards and guidelines for services and treatments; and 3) providing more graduated levels of service to meet consumer demands and thus match need and provision more closely.

Increased investment

There are two broad strategies of increased investment. First, the overall NHS budget and resources devoted to health care will be increased. The UK government has committed itself to an increase in spending of 7.4 per cent per annum in real terms over the financial years 2003/4–2007/8. It is expected that this increase in funding will mean that the NHS's share of the UK's gross domestic product will rise from 7.7 per cent to 9.4 per cent (Robinson 2002). In terms of manpower it is intended that 2,000 extra GPs will be recruited and over 3,000 GP premises will be upgraded (Department of Health 2000a). At a hospital level it is planned to train 7,500 additional consultants, 20,000 extra nurses and 6,500 extra therapists, and to have 7,000 extra beds: around 2,000 for acute care and around 5,000 for intermediate care (at the time of the NHS Plan, the total number of beds on general, acute, and maternity wards was around 147,000 (Department of Health 2000b)). It is also proposed to reduce the time spent by consultants in private practice by awarding a 20 per cent increase in salary for full-time NHS consultants who work full-time for the NHS. Second, additional resources are targeted on particular areas. For example, in April 1999 £20 million from the Modernisation Fund was earmarked for reducing waiting lists and waiting times by enabling 140 NHS Trusts to implement 160 schemes, involving the expansion of facilities, new operating theatres and equipment at these hospitals and units. An extra £250 million will also be invested in information technology in 2003/4, with plans to introduce electronic booking of appointments for patient treatment and electronic prescribing of medicines, and to allow greater co-ordination of care and monitoring of local performance

New ways of organising existing services

Under the NHS Plan, existing services will be 'redesigned' and 'modernised'. In primary care, simple approaches to improve the scheduling of appointments are being used to reduce delays and achieve 'access' targets (Murray 2000). Other examples of innovations to be introduced to increase the efficiency and patient acceptability of care include patient booking systems, extended opening hours for diagnostic services, and establishing elective care treatment centres. In addition, National Service Frameworks and other guidelines aim to set standards and improve the quality of care and efficiency of service provision for major causes of cancer, heart disease and mental illness. There are also specific targets for improving access to both primary and secondary care (Figure 5.1).

Booking systems and targets

Booking systems will be used to give patients a specified time and date for their outpatient appointment or elective admission when they are referred to a hospital clinician or identified as needing an elective admission. Booking systems therefore aim to increase patient choice, because patients will be able to select a time that is

Primary care:
- by March 2004 all patients will be able to get an appointment to see a GP within 48 hours and an appointment to see any other primary care professional within 24 hours;
- by the end of 2000 all patients should have 24 hour access to 'NHS Direct'.

Hospital care:
- by the end of 2005, the maximum wait for an outpatient appointment will be 3 months and the maximum wait for inpatient care 6 months;
- by March 2004, 66% of outpatient appointments and inpatient elective admissions will be arranged using booking systems, and this figure will rise to 100% by the end of 2005 (Department of Health 2000);
- by 2004, for patients requiring inpatient care, the delay between arrival at a casualty department and admission should not be more than 4 hours;
- by 2004, overall average waiting times in casualty departments should be 75 minutes (Department of Health 2000);
- by 2004, there will no longer be 'widespread' bed blocking (Department of Health 2000).

Figure 5.1 Access targets

Source: Department of Health (2000).

convenient to them. They also aim to reduce patient uncertainty because individuals will no longer simply be added to a waiting list and be unclear about when they will gain access to care (Department of Health 2000a). Booking systems also aim to improve the efficient planning of services for elective care. This is because hospital managers will need to ensure that there is adequate capacity to meet scheduled demand. In theory, emergency patients will no longer be able to 'borrow' beds if they have been reserved for booked admissions.

Results from sites which have piloted booking systems for inpatient and day case care indicate that this innovation can lead to reductions in the number of patients waiting for admission, the number of 'do not attends' on an agreed date, and in the number of patient-initiated cancellations (Kipping *et al.* 2000). Unless overall demands for elective care rise, there will be a direct relationship between the first effect and average patient waiting times for care. The latter two effects will help to ensure that existing capacity for elective care is not 'wasted' and hence that the maximum number of patients are treated within existing resources. Results from the pilot sites also indicate that patients (Kipping *et al.* 2000) and hospital doctors (Department of Health 2000a) have positive attitudes to booking systems.

Although the results from these pilot sites are promising, a number of issues will need to be tackled as booking systems are rolled out to a broader number of specialties and hospital sites. A key issue will surround the ease with which the hospital capacity required to meet booked demand can be predicted and scheduled. Consider a booked admission for a hip replacement. As part of their care, patients may need to have access to hospital beds and theatres, services for rehabilitation, and to services to facilitate their acute discharge and for their on-going care in the community. If the right amount of capacity is not available at the right time, delays and inefficiencies will occur.

This matching of capacity and booked demand tends to be easier for day case admissions because most of the key resources are located within dedicated facilities (Kipping *et al.* 2000). It is more difficult when inpatient admissions are booked because the capacity inputs required are likely to be more variable, used over longer time horizons, and spread across more departments both within and beyond the hospital.

Results from the sites that have piloted booking systems (Kipping *et al.* 2000) indicate that the difficulties in matching demand and capacity are greatest for specialties with a high proportion of emergency admissions (because such admissions may 'borrow' capacity that was previously allocated to elective cases). It is also difficult when there is a high degree of variability in the lengths of stay of patients within groupings. A study by Gallivan *et al.* (2002) simulated a booked admission programme for patients requiring cardiac surgery, and in particular the planning and scheduling of beds for intensive care. They concluded that fluctuations in patient stay would cause delays and cancellations if 'reserve' bed capacity was not available. In their simulation, this 'reserve' capacity represented 30 per cent of that which would be needed if all patients' stays corresponded to the mean.

Clinicians have also expressed concerns that direct booking may lead to an increase in referrals from GPs. This concern is being addressed by research being conducted by staff from the University of Birmingham (Meredith *et al.* 2000). Regardless of any changes in overall demand, it will be important to ensure that 'appropriate' patients are offered an outpatient appointment or hospital admission, and that the date which they are offered reflects their need for, and ability to benefit from, treatment.

Other targets for change include waiting times, with the aim that by 2004 patients will have a GP appointment within 48 hours and a maximum wait of three months for an outpatient appointment and six months for an inpatient appointment. Shorter target times for hospital outpatient appointments have also been introduced for suspected cancer, with a two-week target for outpatient review.

Extended opening hours

The current opening hours of hospital departments, such as radiology, which provide information to support the diagnosis and assessment of patients are also seen as a cause of extended acute stay and of 'avoidable' admission to acute care (Department of Health 2001a). Such departments traditionally do not offer a full service, 24 hours a day, seven days a week. Hence, given that hospitals and hospital accident and emergency departments are open 24 hours a day, during the hours when diagnostic departments are not offering a full service, delays in the supply of information to support patient care are likely to occur. As a result, hospitals are being encouraged to develop plans for increasing access to hospital diagnostic departments (Department of Health 2001a). Changes to be considered will include the extension of opening hours (to 24 hours, seven days a week where appropriate) and the increased use of new technologies for 'near patient testing'.

The relevance of, and economic justification for, this policy will vary by hospital. Initially, health care professionals will need to generate information to quantify the extent to which the limited opening hours of diagnostic departments contribute to delays in hospital accident and emergency departments, avoidable admissions to acute care, and/or extended lengths of hospital stay for acute inpatients. For auditing avoidable admissions and delays in acute stay, criteria-based screening tools are available. These tools provide a means of quantifying levels of 'appropriate' and 'avoidable' acute bed use, and for exploring the factors which are leading to 'avoidable' use of beds. Screening tools that have been used in the NHS include the Appropriateness Evaluation Protocol (AEP) (Gertman and Restuccia 1981; O'Neill and Pearson 1995), the Intensity Severity Discharge Adult criteria (ISDA) (Jacobs and Lamprey 1992; Coast *et al.* 1996), and the Oxford Bed Study Instrument (OBSI) (Anderson *et al.* 1988; Fenn *et al.* 2000). The AEP and ISDA are thought to be superior in terms of their validity and reliability (Strumwasser *et al.* 1990) and an adaptation of the AEP is now available for use in NHS hospitals (Bristow *et al.* 1997); the original version of the AEP was developed in the United States. Having quantified the scale of current 'problems', local health care professionals will then need to assess the merits of extending the opening hours of diagnostic departments. The additional investment must be balanced against any expected benefits in terms of reduced delays and patient stay.

Elective care diagnostic and treatment centres

These centres are intended to be independent units devoted solely to the supply of elective care. They aim to increase organisational efficiency by separating 'the bulk of routine elective care from competing emergency pressures' (Department of Health 2001b: 9) thus avoiding the delays and cancellations caused by emergency patients 'borrowing' elective capacity. The target set out in the NHS Plan is that by 2004 eight such centres will be fully developed and will be treating around 200,000 patients per annum, and that a further 12 will be under development.

These centres will treat NHS patients but they will be developed in conjunction with the private sector (Department of Health 2000a). This partnership between the NHS and private providers is part of a more general policy drive whereby NHS commissioners and providers are being encouraged to consider the use of private hospitals as a means of increasing capacity for elective care. As a result, between April and September 2001, contracts were agreed for treating around 29,000 NHS elective patients in private hospitals (Department of Health 2001b).

The implementation of elective care diagnostic and treatment centres is still at a formative stage and evidence of their impacts is still to emerge. A key issue will be whether these centres, and other initiatives which contract out elective care and separate it from emergency workload, affect the 'efficient' supply of services for emergency care. Traditionally adjustments in the admission and work-up of elective patients have been used to accommodate the peaks and troughs of demands for emergency care. Whilst this policy has had undesirable consequences (for example, cancellations and delays in elective care) it has also created a 'reserve' capacity for emergency admissions that could be accessed when required. Such 'reserve' capacity for emergency admissions will still need to be maintained when the option of using capacity for elective care no longer exists. Research indicates that when hospital occupancy rates exceed 85 per cent, hospitals face rapidly increasing difficulties in responding to fluctuations in demands for admission (Bagust et al. 1999; NHS Executive 1998). The importance of adhering to these research findings will increase as the policy of separating emergency and elective care unfolds.

New graduated levels of service

A current aim is to reduce demands on general practice and hospital services by increasing the availability of alternative community-based services, thus increasing the appropriateness and efficiency of service use. Major innovations are the introduction of telephone advice lines, walk-in centres and other nurse-run services at a primary care level, and the development of services for intermediate care as a means of reducing levels of avoidable acute bed use.

Telephone advice lines

A major initiative has been the setting up of NHS Direct as a national 24-hour help line via the telephone. Under this system, nurses, supported by clinical decision support software, provide advice to individuals about the management of their condition and, where required, direct them to the most appropriate health care setting to meet their needs (for example, GP practice or hospital accident and emergency department).

In terms of addressing the difficulties that individuals face in gaining access to health services, NHS Direct aims to offer both quicker access to care and access to care 'out of hours'. In terms of organisational efficiency, this innovation is aiming to ensure that individuals access services at a level and in a setting appropriate to their health care needs. In some instances, it is argued, use of 'traditional' primary care services will be avoided either because telephone advice is sufficient or because individuals are immediately directed to alternative services.

The first wave of NHS Direct sites was evaluated in a study undertaken by staff from the University of Sheffield (Munro and Nichol 1998; Munro et al. 2000). The results indicated that during the first year of the service a population of 1.3 million generated 68,500 calls to NHS Direct: around 72 per cent of these calls were outside the opening hours of 'traditional' GP practices. This incidence of out-of-hours calls (approximately 38 per 1,000 patients) is lower than estimates derived from a study by Salisbury *et al.* (2000) (159 per 1,000 patients). However, this crude comparison does indicate that NHS Direct is meeting a reasonable proportion of demand for out-of-hours care: indeed, the results of the evaluation indicated that there had been a slight reduction in demand for care from GP co-operatives. The proportion of individuals who seek out-of-hours care from NHS Direct may increase as population awareness of this service grows.

The Sheffield evaluation also assessed consumer satisfaction with the service offered by NHS Direct. Levels of satisfaction were high with 97 per cent of respondents indicating that they were 'generally satisfied' and 64 per cent that the service could not be improved. High satisfaction ratings were repeated in a more recent study by the National Audit Office (The Comptroller and Auditor General 2002). However, the report by the National Audit Office (The Comptroller and Auditor General 2002) indicated that although around 60 per cent of the population are aware of NHS Direct, some groups within the population are either unaware of it or unwilling to use it. These include ethnic minority groups, disadvantaged social groups, people with disabilities, young people, and people over 65. Initiatives to try and engage these groups are currently being developed.

The National Audit Office report also noted that nurses tend to exercise a cautious approach in giving advice to callers. This may be because of concerns about the safety and reliability of advice offered via the telephone and the fear that individuals may not be directed to a care setting appropriate to their needs (Nichol and Munro 2000). This may mean that individuals who would be eligible for self-care will be 'unnecessarily' referred to GPs or other health care professionals (George 2002). Uncertainty also surrounds the impact that NHS Direct might have on the continuity of patient care (Nichol and Munro 2000). Again, as the service evolves, there will be a need to ensure that there is an adequate flow of information between all professionals responsible for patient care to ensure patients continuity of care as they access different parts of the system. There are also questions of the impact that NHS Direct may have on the overall demand for health care (Nichol and Munro 2000). There is a fear that this service innovation may generate new demands for health care as well as providing an alternative means of meeting existing demand. Results from the Sheffield evaluation indicated that NHS Direct had a neutral effect on overall demands for health care but again this finding will need to be monitored over time. In addition there is a need to monitor the appropriateness of advice and referrals and the impacts that this service has on health outcomes.

NHS walk-in centres

These centres offer access to advice and treatment for minor conditions without the need for a prior appointment. They are nurse-led but can provide access to general practitioner care if required. Walk-in centres are open for longer hours than 'traditional' general practices, including weekends, and can be based in a range of settings including shops, health centres and hospitals (Salisbury *et al.*

2002). By the end of 2001, 42 of these centres had opened throughout England (Department of Health 2001b). Again, this innovation is aiming to provide individuals with quicker and more convenient access to services for primary care and to improve organisational efficiency by directing patients to a level of care appropriate to their needs.

Government statistics indicate that 100,000 individuals per month used walk-in centres during 2001 (Department of Health 2001b). Based upon this measure of outcome, some centres appear more 'successful' than others. A study by Salisbury *et al.* (2002), of the first 39 walk-in centres to open in the NHS, found that the number of attendances per month by centre ranged from 1,004 to 4,041. Such variations and uncertainties about likely demand create problems when planning the introduction of such services. Without a knowledge of the likely levels and characteristics of demand it is difficult to determine how much, and what type of, capacity should be supplied in walk-in centres: too much and the supply of care will be inefficient and have higher costs than necessary, too little and 'waits' for care will occur.

Considering the characteristics of users of walk-in centres, Salisbury *et al.* (2002) found that young adults represented the highest proportion of users whilst demand from older individuals was comparatively low. Interestingly, levels of demand outside normal working hours was relatively low, indicating that at present the main perceived benefit for users is that these centres provide more convenient access to care than making an appointment to visit a GP. The study by Salisbury *et al.* (2002) found that 78 per cent of patients could have their care needs met within the centre without the need for follow-on referral to another health care professional; individuals most commonly attended because of viral illnesses, for emergency contraception, because of minor injuries, and for the application of dressings. Government publications argue that the demand met by walk-in centres helps to 'free up GPs and A&E Departments to concentrate on more seriously ill or injured patients' (Department of Health 2001b: 7). Salisbury *et al.* (2002) imply that some of the attendances at walk-in centres, particularly amongst young people, represent 'new' demand that might have remained unmet in the past.

Other uncertainties about the impacts of walk-in centres are similar to those which surround NHS Direct. These are: the impacts of walk-in centres on the safety and reliability of care and on the continuity of patient care (Nichol and Munro 2000). Indeed, concerns about variations between centres in the quality of care provided were raised in a study undertaken by the Consumers' Association (Jones 2001).

Intermediate care

The expansion of services for intermediate care is seen as the way of providing alternative care options for those patients for which acute inpatient care is seen as avoidable. Intermediate care services have been defined as those 'designed to prevent avoidable admissions to acute care settings, and to facilitate the transition from hospital to home and from medical dependence to functional independence' (Department of Health 2000c: 13). In addition, a key aim is that, where possible, intermediate care should be delivered in a patient's home or their community (Social Services Inspectorate/NHS Executive 2000).

A range of interventions might fall within the remit of intermediate care. Those highlighted and supported by the NHS plan are:

- multidisciplinary rapid response teams which aim to prevent hospital admission by providing care in a patient's home;
- intensive rehabilitation services to help older patients regain their independence;
- recuperation facilities, using nursing home or other 'step-down' beds for the on-going care of patients who can be discharged from acute care but are not yet ready to go home;
- one-stop clinics for older people to facilitate rapid access to services for health and social care;
- integrated home care teams to help patients live independently at home following hospital discharge.

Intermediate care services are not, in general, aiming to provide novel forms of care but are aiming to provide existing services for assessment and treatment in a more co-ordinated and rapid manner. These services aim to increase organisational efficiency by providing care in a manner, and in a setting, appropriate to the care needs of patients. They also aim to 'release' acute capacity for those individuals who need acute care and, as a result, address the existing delays in admission.

Existing uncertainties about the impacts of intermediate care schemes mirror their overall aims. Hence, issues that are still to be fully resolved include the impacts that intermediate care services can have on levels of avoidable acute bed use; the relative costs of pre-existing and intermediate modes of care; their effects on the clinical outcomes of care; and the attitudes of patients, and their carers, in relation to care 'close to home' (Department of Health 2000b).

In order to examine current evidence about these uncertainties, a series of systematic reviews of the literature were commissioned as part of the national beds inquiry (Goddard et al. (2000); Luff et al. (2000); Lambert and Arblaster (2000)). Other relevant systematic reviews have been undertaken by Parker et al. (2000) and by Hensher et al. (1999). The authors of these reviews tend to be somewhat guarded in making firm conclusions given that, as yet, intermediate care remains an under-researched area.

The current consensus seems to be that discharge facilitation schemes can successfully reduce acute lengths of stay whilst maintaining clinical outcomes (Goddard et al. (2000); Hensher et al. (1999); Parker et al. (2000)). There is less clarity about the impacts that such schemes might have on the overall costs of care. A shortage of completed studies meant that authors were also unwilling to reach preliminary conclusions about the impacts of intermediate care schemes which aim to reduce avoidable bed use by preventing acute admissions: all agreed that more research of such schemes was needed (Goddard *et al.* (2000); Hensher *et al.* (1999); Lambert and Arblaster (2000); Parker *et al.* (2000)).

Finally, both Parker *et al.* (2000) and Luff *et al.* (2000) agreed that there is currently very little evidence upon which to judge whether or not patients and carers prefer care 'close to home'. Luff *et al.* argued that older patients, the dominant client group for intermediate care schemes, appeared to prefer home-based alternatives to hospital although they also indicated that there may be discrepancies between the views of patients and carers.

The above findings demonstrate that there is an urgent need for continuing research to explore uncertainties surrounding the impacts of intermediate care. Locally, as schemes are introduced, there will also be a need for providers to clarify the care needs of potential users so that services can be tailored to meeting these needs. The review conducted by Goddard *et al.* (2000) demonstrated that the intensity of care provided in the community was a key determinant of the likely success of schemes.

Conclusions

This chapter has described some of the main difficulties that individuals currently face in gaining access to the services provided by the NHS of the UK. These difficulties might be summarised as 'waits' and delays in accessing services for primary care, 'waits' for acute elective appointments and investigations, problems in obtaining acute emergency care, and delays surrounding the subsequent delivery of that care. Such access difficulties are most apparent in the NHS of the UK but many of the types of delays that have been described also exist elsewhere.

Waits and delays can be regarded as symptoms of underlying problems. One is the overall level of funds and resources that have been provided for health care within the NHS. This has led to organisational difficulties and rationing to balance supply and demand, through both explicit and less formal mechanisms (see Chapter 11). It is now accepted that this has been insufficient and, as a result, the UK government has committed itself to a rapid, and real terms, increase in spending on the NHS. A second relates to organisational problems affecting the efficiency with which NHS services have traditionally been delivered. These inefficiencies have accentuated the access difficulties that individuals have experienced: either services have been provided at a level that does not match the care needs of patients (for example, care in an acute hospital for patients with sub-acute needs); or services have not been fully utilised (for example, operating theatre sessions are often cancelled).

This chapter has described some of the main service developments and innovations that will be introduced as part of the NHS plan. Preliminary findings indicate that these developments and innovations will have a positive impact on patient access to care, and they may have relevance for other health care systems. Questions remain about both the best ways of implementing these schemes and their wider impacts on the health service. For example, will new primary care services be used in addition to GP services, leading to a duplication of diagnostic tests and treatments? In an increasingly differentiated system, what are the appropriate roles for different types of staff and how can they be coordinated? Is continuity of care important and how can it be facilitated? What implications do these developments have for disadvantaged groups such as chronically disabled or mentally ill people? What effects will these changes have on professional incentives, interests and workloads which will be an important determinant of 'success'? Continued monitoring and evaluation of service developments will be essential.

References

Anderson, P., Meara, J., Broadhurst, S., Attwood, S., Timbrell, M. and Gatherer, A. (1988) 'Use of hospital beds: a cohort study of admissions to a provincial teaching hospital', *British Medical Journal*, 297: 910–12.

Audit Commission (2002) *Operating Theatres: A Bulletin for Health Bodies*. London: Audit Commission. Available http://www.district-audit.gov.uk/home.html; accessed 20 September 2002.

Bagust, A., Place, M. and Posnett, J.W. (1999) 'Dynamics of bed use in accommodating emergency admissions: stochastic simulation model', *British Medical Journal*, 319: 155–8.

Bristow, A., Hudson, M. and Beech, R. (1997) *Analysing Acute Inpatient Services: The Development and Application of Utilisation Review Tools*. Report prepared for the NHS Executive South East Thames. London: NHS Executive South East Thames.

Coast, J., Inglis, A. and Frankel, S. (1996) 'Alternatives to hospital admission: what are they and who should decide?', *British Medical Journal*, 312: 162–6.

Department of Health (1997) *The New NHS: Modern-dependable*, Cmnd 3807. London: Department of Health.

Department of Health (2000a) *The NHS Plan: A Plan for Investment, A Plan for Reform*. London: The Stationery Office.

Department of Health (2000b) *Shaping the Future NHS: Long Term Planning for Hospitals and Related Services*. Consultation document on the findings of the national beds inquiry – supporting analysis. London: Department of Health. Available http://www. doh.gov.uk/ pub/docs/doh/nationalbedsanalysis.pdf; accessed 20 September 2002.

Department of Health (2000c) *Shaping the Future NHS: Long Term Planning for Hospitals and Related Services*. Consultation document on the findings of the national beds inquiry. London: Department of Health. Available http://www.doh.gov.uk/pub/docs/ doh/nationalbeds.pdf; accessed 20 September 2002.

Department of Health (2001a) *Winter and Emergency Services Team – Reforming Emergency Care: First Steps to a New Approach*. London: Department of Health.

Department of Health (2001b) *NHS Emergency Pressures – Making Progress*. London: Department of Health.

Department of Health (2002) *The NHS Plan – A Progress Report: The NHS Modernisation Board's Annual report 2000–2001*. London: Department of Health. Available http:// www.doh.gov.uk/modernisationboardreport/modernisationboardreport.pdf; accessed 20 September 2002.

Department of Health and Social Security (1983). NHS Management Enquiry: Report (Chairman: Mr R. Griffiths). London: DHSS.

Feacham, R.G.A., Sekhri N.K. and White, K.L. (2002) 'Getting more for their dollar: a comparison of the NHS with California's Kaiser Permanente', *British Medical Journal*, 324: 135–43.

Fellin, G., Apolone, G., Tampieri, A., Bevilacqua, L., Meregalli, G., Minella, C. and Liberati, A. (1995) 'Appropriateness of hospital use: an overview of Italian studies', *International Journal for Quality in Health Care*, 7(3): 219–25.

Fenn, A., Horner, P., Travis, S., Prescott, G., Figg, H. and Bates, T. (2000) 'Inappropriate bed usage in a district general hospital', *Journal of Clinical Excellence*, 1: 221–7.

Foster, P (1983) *Access to Welfare. An Introduction to Welfare Rationing*. London: The Macmillan Press.

Frankel, S. and Faulkner A. (1994) 'The end of the outpatient problem?', *British Medical Journal*, 309: 1308.

Gallivan, S., Utley, M., Treasure, T. and Valencia, O. (2002) 'Booked inpatient admissions and hospital capacity: mathematical modelling study', *British Medical Journal*, 324: 280–2.

George, S. (2002) 'NHS Direct audited', *British Medical Journal*, 324: 558.

Gertman, P.M. and Restuccia, J.D. (1981) 'The Appropriateness Evaluation Protocol: a technique for assessing unnecessary days of hospital care', *Medical Care*, 19: 855–71.

Goddard, M., McDonagh, M. and Smith, D. (2000) 'Avoidable use of beds and cost-effectiveness of care in alternative locations'. In Department of Health (2000b) *Shaping the Future NHS: Long Term Planning for Hospitals and Related Services*. Consultation document on the findings of the national beds inquiry – supporting analysis (annex e). London: Department of Health. Available http://www.doh.gov.uk/pub/docs/doh/nationalbedsanalysis.pdf; accessed 20 September 2002.

Hensher, M., Fulop, N., Coast, J. and Jefferys, E. (1999) 'Better out than in? Alternatives to acute hospital care', *British Medical Journal*, 319: 1127–30.

Jacobs, C.M. and Lamprey, J. (1992) *The ISD-A Review System with Adult ISD Criteria*. North Hampton: Interqual.

Jones, J. (2001) 'NHS walk-in centres fail to assess patients properly', *British Medical Journal*, 322: 70.

Kipping, R., Meredith, P., McLeod, H. and Ham, C. (2000) *Booking Patients for Hospital Care: A Progress Report*. Second interim report from the evaluation of the national booked admissions programme. University of Birmingham: Health Services Management Centre.

Lambert, M. and Arblaster, L. (2000) 'Factors associated with acute use of hospital beds by older people: a systematic review of the literature'. In Department of Health (2000b) *Shaping the Future NHS: Long Term Planning for Hospitals and Related Services*. Consultation document on the findings of the national beds inquiry – supporting analysis (annex g). London: Department of Health. Available http://www.doh.gov.uk/pub/docs/doh/nationalbedsanalysis.pdf; accessed 20 September 2002.

Lorenzo, S. and Sunol, R. (1995) 'An overview of Spanish studies on appropriateness of hospital use', *International Journal for Quality in Health Care*, 7(3): 213–8.

Luff, D., Nicholl, J., O'Cathain, A., Munro, J. and Paisley, S. (2000) 'Patient preferences'. In Department of Health (2000b) *Shaping the Future NHS: Long Term Planning for Hospitals and Related Services*. Consultation document on the findings of the national beds inquiry – supporting analysis (annex f). London: Department of Health. Available http://www.doh.gov.uk/pub/docs/doh/nationalbeds analysis.pdf; accessed 20 September 2002.

Malbon, G., Jenkins, C. and Gillam, S. (2000) *What do Londoners Think of Their General Practice?* London: King's Fund.

Mays, N. (1997) 'Origins and development of the National Health Service'. In G. Scambler (ed) *Sociology as Applied to Medicine.* London: W.B. Saunders.

McDonagh, M.S., Smith, D.H. and Goddard, M. (2000) 'Measuring appropriate use of acute beds: a systematic review of methods and results', *Health Policy*; 53: 157–84.

McKee, M. and Waghorn, A. (2000) 'Why is it so difficult to organise an outpatient clinic?', *Journal of Health Services Research and Policy*, 5(3): 140–7.

McKinley, R.K., Cragg, D.K., Hastings, A.M., French, D.P., Manku-Scott, T.K., Campbell, S.M., Van, F., Roland, M.O. and Roberts, C. (1997) 'Comparison of out of hours care provided by patients' own general practitioners and commercial deputising services: a randomised controlled trial II: the outcome of care', *British Medical Journal*, 314: 190–3.

Meredith, P., Ham, C. and Kipping, R. (2000) *Modernising the NHS: Booking Patients for Hospital Care – A Progress Report.* First interim report from the evaluation of the national booked admissions programme. University of Birmingham: Health Services Management Centre.

Munro, J. and Nicholl, J. (1998) *Evaluation of NHS Direct First Wave Sites: First Interim Report to the Department of Health.* University of Sheffield: Medical Care Research Unit.

Munro, J., Nicholl, J., O'Cathain, A. and Knowles, E. (2000) 'Impact of NHS Direct on demand for immediate care: observational study', *British Medical Journal*, 321: 150–3.

Murray, M. (2000) 'Patient care: access', *British Medical Journal*, 320: 1594–6.

NHS Executive (1998) *Second report of the Emergency Services Action Team* (ESAT). Leeds: NHS Executive.

NHS Executive West Midlands (1998) *The Rise in Admissions Project: A Report to the West Midland NHS Executive.* A report prepared by Coventry Business School, Coventry University, Department of Health Sciences and Clinical Evaluation and York Health Economics Consortium, University of York, Office of the Vice-Chancellor, Plymouth University. Birmingham: NHS Executive West Midlands.

Nicholl, J. and Munro, J. (2000) 'Systems for emergency care: integrating the components is the challenge', *British Medical Journal*, 320: 955–6.

O'Neill, D. and Pearson, M. (1995) 'Appropriateness of hospital use in the United Kingdom: a review of activity in the field', *International Journal of Quality in Health Care*, 7(3): 239–44.

Packwood, T., Keen, J. and Buxton, M. (1991) *Hospitals in Transition: The Resource Management Experiment.* Milton Keynes: Open University Press.

Parker, G., Bhakta, P., Katbamna, S., Lovett, C., Paisley, S., Parker, S., Phelps, K., Baker, R., Jagger, C., Lindsay, J., Shepperdson, B. and Wilson, A. (2000) 'Best place of care for older people after acute and during sub acute illness: a systematic review', *Journal of Health Services Research and Policy*, 5(3): 176–89.

Pickin, M., Sampson, F., Munro, J. and Nicholl, J. (2001) 'General practitioners' reasons for removing patients from their lists: postal survey in England and Wales', *British Medical Journal*, 322: 1158–9.

Pope, C. (1991) 'Trouble in store: some thoughts on the management of waiting lists', *Sociology of Health and Illness*, 13(2): 193–212.

Robinson, R. (2002) 'Gold for the NHS: good news that raises questions on consistency and sustainability', *British Medical Journal*, 324: 987–8.

Salisbury, C., Trivella M. and Bruster, S. (2000) 'Demand for and supply of out of hours care from general practitioners in England and Scotland: observational study based on routinely collected data', *British Medical Journal*, 320: 618–21.

Salisbury, C., Chalder, M., Scott, T.M., Pope, C. and Moore, L. (2002) 'What is the role of walk-in centres in the NHS?', *British Medical Journal*, 324: 399–402.

Scrivens, E., Cropper, S. and Beech, R. (1999) *Making Winter Monies Work: A Review of Locally Used Methods for Selecting and Evaluating Supply-side Interventions*. Keele: Keele University, Centre for Health Planning and Management. Available http://www.keele.ac.uk/depts/hm/chpmhmpg.htm; accessed 20 September 2002.

Secretaries of State for Health, Wales, Northern Ireland and Scotland (1989) *Working for Patients*, Cmnd 555. London: HMSO.

Social Services Inspectorate/NHS Executive (2000) *Millennium Executive Team Report on Winter 1999/2000*. London: Department of Health.

Strumwasser, I., Paranjipe, N., Ronis, D., Share, D. and Sell, L.J. (1990) 'Reliability and validity of utilisation review criteria', *Medical Care*, 28(2): 95–111.

Teale, G.R., Moffitt, D.D., Mann, C.H. and Luesley, D.M. (2000) 'Management guidelines for women with normal colposcopy after low grade cervical abnormalities: population study', *British Medical Journal*, 320: 1693–6.

The Comptroller and Auditor General (2002) *NHS Direct in England*. London: The Stationery Office.

Wanless, D. (2002) *Securing Our Future Health: Taking a Long Term View*. London: The Public Enquiry Unit, HM Treasury.

World Health Organisation Regional Office for Europe, European Stroke Council (1995) *Pan European Consensus Meeting on Stroke Management*. Helsingborg: World Health Organisation.

Worthington, D. (1997) 'Queue management: what has a DSS approach to offer to improve the running of outpatient clinics?'. In S. Cropper and P. Forte (eds) *Enhancing Decision Making in the NHS: The Role of Decision Support Systems*. Buckingham: Open University Press.

Chapter 6

Financial incentives and barriers to access

David Hughes

Introduction

Financial barriers to health care are important at the level of the health system, the organisation, and the individual. At the health system level, the availability of services is determined by the total amount of resources allocated to health care, and by the distribution of resources to different types of service and to different geographical areas. At the organisational level, different payment methods offer providers incentives that either encourage or discourage the provision and delivery of specific services. At the individual level, financial incentives to patients can either encourage or discourage the consumption of services, thus acting as a barrier or gateway to services. The relevance of financial barriers at these different levels varies according to the organisation, and methods of financing, of the health system. In the UK, the NHS was established with the aim of removing personal financial barriers to accessing health care. However, the NHS is financed centrally from general taxation and there has been increasing concern that this central control of health care funding has itself limited access to health care. Choice of provider is also restricted in the UK except for those who are willing or able to pay for private care. These arrangements are in marked contrast to the situation in the US where personal financial barriers are of great importance, but there is almost unrestricted access and choice for those who are able to pay.

This chapter begins with a discussion of financing and rationing of health care. It goes on to discuss the impact of financial barriers and incentives on the behaviour of patients and providers in both primary care and secondary care. The subject of resource allocation is discussed in Chapter 2. The relevance of financial barriers to access in the United States and in the European Union is discussed in Chapters 7 and 8 respectively.

Financing of health care

A number of different approaches have been employed to determine whether the level of health care funding in the UK is appropriate (Dixon *et al.* 1997). An economic approach, which relates the potential benefits of increases in service provision to their costs, is difficult to apply. The political debate has therefore been dominated by negative public perceptions of access to health care, and by unfavourable international comparisons of health care funding (Dixon *et al.* 1997). Public perceptions have been shaped by a series of incidents in which individual patients failed to gain access to services such as intensive care beds (Parmanum *et al.* 2000), the continuing problems of long waiting lists and waiting times, and other problems with the quality of services (see Chapter 5). Examples include well-publicised adverse incidents in cardiac surgical (Pande 1998) and cancer screening and treatment services (Tobias 1988). Professional perceptions have also been influenced by a series of studies which showed that UK patients with treatable conditions such as breast cancer have worse health outcomes than in other European countries. In the period 1985–9, the five-year survival rate for breast cancer was 67 per cent in England compared with rates of approximately 80 per cent in France and Sweden (Quinn *et al.* 1998).

Against a background of difficulties in accessing services of adequate quality, it is clear that overall health care funding in the UK has lagged behind that of other OECD countries. Table 6.1 shows the total health care expenditure in several OECD countries (Wanless 2001). Health expenditure in the UK represents a low proportion of GDP, and the overall level of health expenditure is low compared with the other countries. The UK also has one of the smallest private health care sectors. The UK government acknowledged these problems and published the national NHS Plan whose overall aims were to increase access to health care by increasing health service capacity, and by modernising and redesigning services so as to remove organisational barriers to access (Department of Health 2000) (see Chapter 5). An independent report commissioned by the UK Treasury endorsed a new consensus that health care funding in the UK was inadequate and suggested that government health care expenditure should increase from UK£68 billion in 2002 to between UK£154 and UK£184 billion in 2022–3 (in 2002–3 prices) (Wanless 2002). The precise estimate required depended on the assumptions made about the changing health of the population. It was estimated that health care spending would account for 9.4 per cent of GDP by 2008 (Wanless 2002). Another important conclusion from the Wanless report (Wanless 2001), was the confirmation that financing from taxation was considered to provide the fairest method for funding health care (Wagstaff and van Doorslaer 1992; Wagstaff *et al.* 1999) .

Rationing

Rationing decisions

While the UK National Health Service is a cash limited system, there is a problem of almost unlimited demand due to the nature of health care and the definition of ill health, which keeps changing as technology advances. Increasing demands for health care mean that access to diagnosis and treatment is rationed. One definition

Table 6.1 Health expenditure per capita and as a percent of GDP (1998)

Country	Total health care expenditure (US$ per capita)	Percent of GDP		
		Total	Public	Private
USA	4,165	12.9	5.8	7.1
Germany	2,361	10.3	7.8	2.5
Canada	2,360	9.3	6.5	2.8
Netherlands	2,150	8.7	6.0	2.7
Australia	2,085	8.6	6.0	2.6
France	2,034	9.3	7.1	2.2
Japan	1,795	7.4	5.8	1.6
Sweden	1,732	7.9	6.6	1.3
UK	1,510	6.8	5.7	1.1
New Zealand	1,440	8.1	6.3	1.9

Source: Wanless (2001).

suggests that rationing represents 'societal toleration of inequitable access to health services' (Hadorn 1991).

That resources are scarce and so must be rationed is indisputable. The question is not whether all individuals should be able to access all services but, rather, who should be restricted from accessing certain services and which services should be provided within the health care system. Rationing decisions are made in many different contexts and at many different levels. Wherever resources are rationed, access is restricted.

This may involve restricting access to specific services for certain groups, due to their characteristics, such as their age or type of condition, or implicitly through the notion of opportunity cost, whereby some services are delivered at the expense of others because resources simply run out. For example, public sector funding of nursing home care for older people is currently severely restricted in England and Wales (Christie 2002).

In order to achieve the aims of the health care system, decisions should be made on an explicit basis. The UK government recently established the National Institute for Clinical Excellence (NICE) whose role is to provide patients, health professionals and the public with authoritative guidance on current 'best practice'. Guidance covers both individual health technologies (including medicines, medical devices, diagnostic techniques, and procedures) and the clinical management of specific conditions. NICE develops clinical guidelines to help health professionals deliver care which is more clinically effective and cost-effective, and rationing decisions are more explicit.

Some of the decisions made by NICE have already filtered through into service delivery. For example, sildenafil (Viagra), a new treatment for erectile dysfunction, is being made available on the NHS only to people who have specifically identified conditions which cause erectile dysfunction. Other judgements have been made on beta-interferon, and anti-psychotic and anti-cancer drugs. The implications for access are clear. Some individuals are prevented from gaining access to health care as a result of their characteristics, or the nature and cause of their disease, or through their own behaviour. Other treatments are not provided through the publicly funded health service although they may be available privately. For example only around 18 per cent of all in vitro fertilisation (IVF) treatments are provided through the NHS, which creates a potential inequity of access related to ability to pay.

Rationing principles

Ideally, resources should be allocated according to the objectives of the health service, taking into account the benefits and costs of treatments. Health services may have several potential objectives including, for example, increasing health gain, or minimising health inequalities. In reality, objectives will be multiple and conflicting. Even if it were possible to narrow the objectives down to 'improving health', many different groups might be given priority. New (1996) suggested that the health service might focus on improving the health of specific groups of people including those most in need (those with greatest ill health), particular disadvantaged groups (poor, ethnic minorities), people upon whom others depend (those with children) or particular age groups (those who have most of their lives before them). If the objective is to maximise health benefits, then resources should be allocated to those patients or groups who will benefit most for a given use of resources.

The measurement of benefits is a highly contentious issue. The assessment of benefit might be measured on a range of dimensions including personal benefits, in term of mortality, health-related quality of life, and satisfaction, but also by less tangible factors such as autonomy, moral worth and dignity. There is general consensus that the benefits of health care should at least take into account two key dimensions: length and quality of life. It is often argued that those treatments that extend length of life by the longest, holding all other factors equal, should be favoured over those which extend life by a lesser amount. This of course has serious implications for individual comparisons; it will, for example, favour the young over the elderly. There is evidence to suggest that this may reflect societal values (Bowling 1996).

If we take account of the outcome of health care intervention in terms of length of life, individuals who are likely to benefit over a longer period of their life should get priority for resources. As indicated above, this would have implications for groups such as the elderly, but may also affect other groups, such as smokers. For example, the prognosis for smokers after coronary artery bypass grafting is worse than for non-smokers, as life expectancy and often quality of life are lower than for the equivalent non-smoker. It is sometimes argued that since smokers inflict self-harm, they are less deserving. The implications of these decisions are not trivial; if we extrapolate these decisions to other groups we could argue that other groups who put themselves at risk are less deserving, for example individuals who undertake dangerous sports.

Some commentators support these implications but others reject rationing along these lines. The rejection of rationing on the basis of age (and implicitly rationing with the aim of maximising health care benefits) is usually on the basis of notions of social justice and equity. The egalitarian notion that like patients should be treated equally, and unlike patients unequally, is strongly based within the National Health Service. The implications for access to health care are important but there is little consensus regarding the over-riding principle of whether a concern for equity or efficiency should predominate (Sassi *et al.* 2001).

The notion of efficiency in the context of rationing health care is seen as an ethical choice concerned with maximising improvements in health for the population as a whole. Cost, particularly the notion of opportunity cost, is central to the rationing decision. Every decision to treat one individual, or group of individuals, involves a loss to another group which remains untreated. Cost is an underlying constraint on all the objectives of the NHS. The cost of treatments and the sacrifice made by groups who forgo treatments is central to the whole issue of access.

Rationing involves consideration of both efficiency (benefit) and equity (fairness) in deciding allocation criteria, and recognition of the trade-off between the two. If equity of access is considered to be the over-riding principle determining resource allocation then we must accept that benefits will not be maximised. An integrated rationing process requires management of the criteria for patient access to the health care system.

Rationing in practice

In reality, individuals who make rationing decisions do not have the time or the information to be able to make fully informed decisions based on the total needs of the population. The health care system may also offer incentives to providers to deliver certain services or to restrict access for certain groups of service users. Many decisions concerning who to treat are based on ad hoc decision-making which can lead to arbitrary variations in access to health care. As long as rationing decisions are made in a covert and implicit way, access to health care will be variable, the aims of the health care system will not be fully met, and a proper debate about efficiency and equity will not be possible.

Financial incentives and service providers

Financial incentives to service providers can influence both the quantity and the type of services available. Payments to general practitioners (GPs) for specific services such as immunisation and screening can result in their being more willing to provide these services. If this happens, then access to secondary care may be reduced because primary physicians have an incentive to provide care and may be more reluctant to refer patients to hospitals. Hospitals themselves receive payments for providing different types of services, and these payments create incentives that influence the provision and delivery of services and thus the number of patients having access to treatment.

Offering a financial incentive to provide services should not be considered to be intrinsically wrong. If incentives can be used to achieve public policy goals, then these may be the best way of encouraging the provision of a particular service and may improve access to care. As Lu and Donaldson (2000) recognised, incentive payments can increase health care outputs including access, quantity and effectiveness as well as reducing costs of care. Payments introduce complex incentives to providers, which makes the evaluation of the effect of payments on health care systems a challenging task.

Paying general practitioners

In the UK, general medical practitioners (GPs) are paid through a mix of capitation allowances and fee-for-service payments, together with additional sessional payments and target payments for providing particular services and achieving certain predetermined levels of service (for a detailed literature review of studies estimating the impact of these types of payments see Gosden *et al.* (2000)). The reform of GPs' remuneration in the UK in the early 1990s aimed to make general practice more responsive to consumers' wishes and change the emphasis from treatment to prevention by using financial incentives. More recently, GPs have been increasingly offered salaried status in order to attract them to practice in under-served areas.

Capitation payments

Capitation payments are payments received by GPs for each patient on their list. One main advantage of the capitation method of payment is that it provides GPs with an incentive to encourage patients to join, and remain on, their list and to be responsive to their patients' needs and demands (Donaldson and Gerrard 1989). Another advantage claimed for the capitation system is that it is consistent with the independent status of the GP. That is, it provides minimal interference with medical judgement and, potentially at least, provides a link between the income of the GP and his or her workload – represented by the list size. GPs may respond to a larger list size by reducing the length of consultations (Campbell *et al.* 2001), although this may improve overall access to care (shorter consultations may improve throughput), the quality of care may be diminished.

One of the criticisms of the capitation-based system is that there may be an incentive to attract low-cost patients with a low risk of illness. Capitation payments are only adjusted very crudely for the likely burden to the practice of providing care. Payments are weighted for patient age and the level of deprivation in the enumeration district of residence. The incentive which these payments provide depends on the cost to the practice of providing care to the patient and the level at which the capitation fee is set. If capitation payments to GPs do not cover the full cost of care for certain types of patient then this can limit access to care, as GPs will not be fully reimbursed for care provided (Donaldson 1989). Thus although capitation payments are weighted for deprivation, this may not be sufficient to offset the increased workload and other disadvantages of delivering services in a deprived area (Gravelle and Sutton 1998).

The capitation system may also encourage GPs to minimise their own input into consultations by reducing the length of consultations, prescribing more, or referring more patients to hospital. A study by Krasnik *et al.* (1990) in Denmark, which investigated the effects on GPs' activities of changing from a wholly capitation-based payment system to a mixed fee-per-item and capitation system, found evidence to support this. The authors concluded that general practitioners whose remuneration was capitation-based, and therefore not directly linked to workload, were more likely to refer patients to the hospital sector. This may affect access to hospitals by creating extra demand for services and has implications for appropriateness of care. Hughes and Yule (1991) suggested that GPs may find it less easy to respond to incentives linked to list size, since they may only have limited control over the number of patients on their list. This questions the overall effectiveness of capitation payments as a means of influencing GPs' behaviour.

Per-item fees

In the UK, GPs are paid fees for providing particular items of service such as immunisations. Per-item fees have the advantage of rewarding GPs according to the amount of work they carry out, and these can be used to encourage GPs to provide specific services. Per-item fees have been criticised as a method of payment because they may encourage GPs to recommend services to patients that will have little or no beneficial impact on the health of the patient, but will remunerate the practitioner. The extent to which physicians induce demand for their services has received attention in several North American studies. Donaldson and Gerard (1992) concluded that much of the evidence is ambiguous. Some of the North American studies found strong evidence that the amount of care provided by GPs (or primary care physicians in the US) is influenced by the level of payments. For example, Rice (1983) found that decreasing the reimbursement rate by 1 per cent resulted in an increase of 0.61 per cent in service intensity, and a 1 per cent decrease in the reimbursement rate for surgical services resulted in a 0.15 per cent increase in service intensity. This suggests that physicians may respond to changes in fee levels, at least in the US.

Culyer (1989), in a similar review, concluded that fee-for-service methods result in more active treatment and higher incomes for doctors, although most evidence referred to the US. In a UK-based study, Horder *et al.* (1986) suggested that the existence of per-item payments for cervical cytology was one of the influences leading GPs to increase the total number of smears they carried out by over 400 per cent between 1966 and 1980, although clearly other factors may have influenced this increase, including public awareness and attitudes to smear tests. A study by

Hughes and Yule (1992) employed quantitative techniques to examine the impact that per-item payments had on GPs' use of cervical cytology and maternity care in the UK over the period 1967–89. They found little evidence to suggest that changes in per-item fees were associated with the number of treatments provided.

In a system where the fees are set centrally, as in the UK, the incentive to provide treatments, or induce demand, might depend on the level at which fees are set. If fees are set at such a level that they fail to compensate the GP for the cost of providing the service there may be little incentive to provide the service. Scheffler *et al.* (1996) estimated the 'payment elasticity of access' for dentistry in the US. That is, the proportionate increase in access that occurs for a specific proportionate increase in payment. For Medicaid dental services, the payment elasticity of access was found to be relatively low. While providers increased participation and the level of service they provided, this did not translate into corresponding increases in access. A 10 per cent increase in payment translated into greater dental participation in the Medicaid programme, but yielded less than 1 per cent increase in access. Mayer *et al.* (2000) also suggested that reimbursement rate increases were only marginally effective in increasing access to dental services for the Medicaid population. These results have implications for other public service programmes with access issues and suggest that the level of payment, at least for dentistry, does not substantially affect the level of service.

The impact of payments systems may have differential effects for population groups. Haber and Mitchell (1999) examined whether changes in physician reimbursement under the Medicare Fee Schedule (MFS) had differential impacts on access to care for vulnerable and non-vulnerable patients in the Medicare scheme. The study identified several vulnerable groups including people living in areas that were poor or which had a shortage of health professionals and people who were African American, disabled or very old. The study selected a random sample to ensure adequate representation of vulnerable group members and constructed service-specific measures of the MFS payment change. The authors found that few effects on access were attributable to the MFS. However, they did find substantial utilisation gaps between vulnerable and non-vulnerable sub-populations for primary care services, as well as for high-cost procedures during episodes of care for acute myocardial infarctions.

Target payments and sessional fees

Target payments are flat rate fees that are paid to GPs once they achieve a predetermined level of service such as providing vaccinations for 80 per cent of the children on their list. These payments have the advantage of remunerating GPs directly in line with their workload based on their success in achieving particular levels of services, and, as with per-item fees, can be used to encourage GPs to fulfil public policy goals.

Target payments have the disadvantage that if a GP cannot reach the 'target' level, there is no incentive to provide any care at all. Once the target level is reached there is no incentive to provide any more care over and above this level, which may lead to individuals who could benefit from a service not being catered for, and access being restricted. For example, a target level for coverage for cervical smears set at 80 per cent requires that GPs provide smears for 80 per cent of their list within a predetermined population group. It is not obvious that the 20 per cent they do not screen would not benefit from the service, or that the 80 per cent they do screen are those who would benefit most; therefore, the target levels are in many ways arbitrary.

While the average coverage of the population may be high, this may mask geographical inequities. In some areas GPs may not be able to reach the lower target. Thus, there is no incentive to provide the service since they will not be paid for any services provided below the lower target level. Consequently, service provision may vary between GPs and between regions.

Since target payments are a relatively new form of payment there is, as yet, little evidence regarding the impact of this form of payment. Some of the available evidence suggests that target payments have been effective in increasing provision. Hughes and Yule (1992), using the model they developed to analyse the impact of fees in the period 1967–89, estimated the impact of the introduction of target payments. They found that in the first year of target payments there was a 50 per cent increase in the number of cervical smears carried out by GPs, relative to the level they estimated would have been performed had per-item payments been retained. A recent review of target payments (Giuffrida *et al.* 2000) suggested that the available evidence was 'not of sufficient quality or power' to determine the effectiveness of target payments.

Sessional fees, as with target payments, reward GPs directly in line with the work they carry out. At least in the UK where clinics that provide 'health promotional activities' attract sessional payments, the incentive may be to undertake 'clinics' where previously the work might have been carried out in ordinary consultations. Evidence from a study carried out shortly after the revised GP contract was introduced in 1990 suggested that significantly more patients were being seen by GPs in clinics after the new contract than before (Hannay *et al.* 1992). Consequently, the costs of providing a service may increase without any corresponding increase in health. Sessional payments may, therefore, encourage GPs to over-provide certain activities, regardless of the impact on the health of the patients.

Allowances

Allowances are paid for fulfilling certain requirements, such as providing a minimum number of surgery hours, or operating with a certain minimum practice list size. They have the advantage of providing a stable income and can encourage GPs to fulfil certain policy aims (such as encouraging group practice). They have the potential disadvantage of failing to give GPs a direct incentive to respond to patients' wishes. As with capitation payments, since payment is not linked to workload the incentive may be for GPs to minimise their own workload, although, as with capitation payments, they may be seen to provide minimal interference with medical judgement.

Salaried status

The financial incentives provided by the standard GP contract have typically encouraged GPs to practice in more affluent areas (Gravelle and Sutton 2001). The number of GPs in an area is regulated to some extent through the Medical Practices Committee (MPC) but there remains a substantial imbalance in the geographical distribution of GPs with more deprived areas generally having fewer GPs (Benzeval and Judge 1996). Since 1997 the NHS has allowed the contractual arrangements for GPs to be varied so that local provider organisations were able to offer local service contracts designed to meet the needs of local populations (Williams *et al.* 2001a). These 'primary medical services' (PMS) contracts were mainly designed to encourage GPs to practice in deprived areas which were under-served. Initial evaluations of these schemes have shown that salaried GPs earned less than those employed on standard contracts, but their satisfaction with their contract was similar, and overall they experienced less stress than GPs employed on standard contracts (Gosden *et al.* 2002). These findings might have been explained to some extent by individual GPs choosing their preferred type of contract. However, the findings serve to emphasise the importance of other motivating factors such as the hours of work, the burden of administrative duties, and the availability of opportunities for personal development (Williams *et al.* 2001a; Gosden *et al.* 2002).

Paying hospitals

There are three main methods of reimbursing hospitals: retrospective at full cost, prospective on a per-case basis, or through a market-based system. Each method has potential implications for hospital activity.

Retrospective payments

Retrospective payments systems involve hospitals receiving payment in full for all expenditures incurred during a pre-defined period. This system encourages hospitals to do as much work as possible, or to maximise lengths of stay, and provide as many diagnostic tests and other procedures. Anecdotal evidence from the US suggests that the method of retrospective reimbursement accompanied a period of substantial growth in health care expenditure.

Prospective payments

In contrast, the prospective reimbursement system requires hospitals to provide a service within a given budget. The level of payment received can be based on an estimation of the expected workload, and may be broken down into individual case-based payments. The reimbursement level is then set for each case type and the total budget received is based on how many cases the hospital provides (or is expected to provide). This type of system encourages hospitals to minimise costs by shortening lengths of stay, substituting less costly inputs for more expensive ones, or by reducing the quality of care. Hospitals may be encouraged to 'cost-shift' whereby they shift patients into other sectors rather than incurring the costs of care themselves, for example to long-term care, or to the patient's own home. These actions clearly have implications for access to secondary care facilities. Rosko and Broyles (1987) found that length of stay had shortened under the prospective payment system but a study by Carroll and Erwin (1987) concluded that there was little evidence that cost-shifting from hospital to other settings took place.

As with any payment system, the level at which the payment is set is crucial. Hamilton (1993) examined the implications of fixed-price reimbursement of providers for access to hospice care by Medicare beneficiaries. Hospices that were offered higher reimbursement rates by Medicare were found to be more likely to become certified to provide care under the Medicare Hospice Benefit programme. Each $1.00 increase in the daily routine home care rate raises the probability of certification by 1.7 per cent. In turn, the Hospice Benefit increased access to hospice care by enabling Medicare-certified facilities to serve more patients than they would if they were non-certified. Hamilton pointed out that reimbursement rates must be set appropriately. Failure to correctly adjust reimbursement rates for the real costs of certification across different parts of the country can lead to disparities in hospice certification and differential access to hospice care for Medicare beneficiaries. Glied (1998) suggested that incentives should be designed to reduce risk selection and ensure access to appropriate specialty services. The design of payments systems is important because side effects may include reduced access to 'unprofitable' services.

Prospective payments to reimburse physicians for serving Medicaid patients have been rising in many states in the US. Policy-makers anticipate that higher fees will increase access to services. Travis (1999) explored whether physicians respond to the increased payment by increasing access differentially by patient type. Empirical tests using Medicaid data from 1988 to 1991 for antenatal care provision in Washington State showed that fees are relevant in improving access to care for the average patient, with significantly greater improvement for Hispanics and single patients.

Market-based system

A market-based system allows hospitals to set their own payments levels and to compete for patients. The result of competition may be varied. Hospitals potentially have an incentive to attract patients to their facilities, and this may be achieved through higher-quality care, but they also have an incentive to minimise costs, which may compromise quality. The outcome depends on whether competition takes place predominantly through price or quality. In the US it has been suggested that competition has resulted in a health care style 'arms race' where hospitals compete on the basis of high technology equipment. This may improve access to up-to-date technology and diagnostic aids, but may not promote efficiency across the health system. Regulation of health care markets is required to ensure that provider behaviour is directed towards planned objectives (Saltman 2002).

The logic of the market is such that a situation will arise in which hospitals will have differential provision of services. Some will have insufficient capacity to treat demand, some will have under-utilised capacity, while others may be forced to close. This situation will persist until some sort of equilibrium is reached. Provider markets can promote geographical equity since out-of-area purchases of services may release patients from dependence on locally accessible services (Culyer *et al.* 1988). It is argued that consumer choice may be enhanced through competition, and relative efficiency may be enhanced through market forces. Whether this improves access is an open question. Generally, improvements in efficiency may improve the number of services provided from the available resources, thus allowing overall provision to increase.

User charges and patients' use of services

Financial incentives can influence patients because, although the UK system is essentially 'free at the point of use', charges are made for specific services including eye tests, dental check ups, and dispensing of prescription medicines. In addition to user charges, the indirect costs of accessing care, such as costs of travel and time lost from work may also influence access as discussed in Chapter 2. Charges can act as a deterrent to patients and as a barrier to access. User charges affect different socio-economic groups in different ways. For some groups access may not be compromised by a co-payment, while for others the charge may represent a significant deterrent. The impact depends on the size of the co-payment and crucially depends on patients' ability to pay (and therefore directly links with equity considerations, see Chapter 3). Public funding of health care, and the insurance market, essentially remove most financial barriers to access so that patients do not face the full cost of care. This of course creates an incentive itself, where patients may over-consume services. Where this occurs other patients with more pressing needs may have problems accessing services (waiting times will become longer and patients who require urgent care may be displaced). It is argued that insurance-based systems create a further problem, which is known as 'moral hazard', whereby individuals fail to take full responsibility for their own health as they do not face the full costs of any ill-health associated with their behaviour (for example, smokers might not smoke if they had to pay the full costs for cancer treatment). Thus insurance systems take away barriers to access and this may lead to inappropriate utilisation of services, or may lead to excess demand for services and the subsequent problems this causes with respect to prioritising care.

The impact of user charges, or fees, levied on services is straightforward. If people have to pay for a service they will use less of it. The main impact of user charges is, therefore, on utilisation. The rationale behind user charges is that they can be used to deter inappropriate utilisation of services, raise revenue for the health service and act as a reminder to individuals of the value of the services they consume. There are clearly disadvantages, as user charges can have the negative impact of potentially excluding low-income individuals from consuming beneficial health care services (see Chapter 8 for further discussion).

Many studies have considered the impact of user charges and co-payments. Most research has focused on how cost-sharing affects the use of medical services rather than health outcomes (Rice and Morrison 1994). The RAND Corporation in the US carried out the most complete examination of the impact of user charges on health service use. The experiments evaluated the effect of varying the initial amount of cost-sharing (the amount paid by patients for services) on health service use. They found, not surprisingly, that utilisation of all types of service (physician visits, hospital admissions, prescriptions, dental visits, etc.) fell as cost-sharing increased (Newhouse 1996).

The NHS since its inception has aimed to make health care available to all regardless of income and at the same time assure equitable distribution of resources regionally. Until the reforms introduced by the 1989 White Paper, the NHS was characterised by centralised financing and regulation. There are two main areas where user charges are imposed: dental services and prescription charges. The impact of user charges in these two health care sectors has been examined in the UK.

Hughes and McGuire (1995) estimated the impact of charges for drug prescriptions in the NHS and found evidence to suggest that user charges reduced the number of prescriptions cashed in the UK. The impact of user charges is likely to affect different socio-economic groups differently. Lundberg et al. (1998) found that price sensitivity decreased with age, income, education and self-rated health-status. Sensitivity to user charges for drugs varied greatly between different types of drugs; for example, if user charges doubled they found that 40 per cent of anti-tussive users would reduce their consumption, whereas only 11 per cent of users of drugs for menopausal problems would reduce their consumption. It should be recognised that in the UK user charges are means tested; low-income families and people over 65 years are exempt, as are individuals with certain chronic conditions, such as diabetes.

Recent changes in the NHS General Dental Service have arguably led to a reduction in the availability of NHS dental care and increased charges (see Chapter 9). A study by Stoelwinder (1994) explored public and user views and experiences of NHS and private dental care in the light of these changes. The study employed a combination of quantitative and qualitative methods. The first phase involved a postal survey of a random sample of adults on the electoral registers in a county in southern England. Follow-up face-to-face interviews were carried out with sub-samples selected from survey respondents. The evidence showed greater satisfaction with certain aspects of private care than with NHS dental care and suggested that the decline in perceived quality of NHS care is less to do with the quality of dental technical skills and more to do with access and availability. There was general support for the egalitarian principles associated with NHS dentistry; payment for dental care by users was acceptable, though dentistry on the NHS was preferred. The shift in the balance of NHS and private dental care reflects the interests and preferences of dentists rather than of the public. It suggests that a continued shift towards private practice is a trend that the public will not find acceptable, which might limit the extent of expansion of private practice.

Some commentators suggested that user charges could be extended in the UK. Mufti (2000) suggested that user charges would be an important source of revenue in the United Kingdom where services cannot be cut and tax increases are politically risky. He argued that user charges in public facilities would curtail over-utilisation and reduce inefficient use of resources by providing a link between financial responsibility and the provision of services. The financial implication facing patients would encourage them to be more cost-conscious, and their physicians would be encouraged to limit over-prescribing of drugs and the use of highly specialised diagnostic procedures for routine investigation or minor illnesses. Mufti suggested that the lack of economic incentives has led to a lack of concern for the cost of medical care. User charges would not only encourage both consumers and providers to be cost-conscious, but would also raise revenue to ease pressure on the health budget, combat moral hazards and assert priorities. In order to be effective and make a serious impact on the health system, Mufti argued that user charges must be extended to all government sectors and specialist hospitals and charges must be high enough to discourage inappropriate use of services. However, as we noted earlier, concerns for equity do not support these arguments (Wagstaff and van Doorslaer 1992; Wagstaff et al. 1999).

The role of the private sector

The influence of user charges on patients' use of services is particularly relevant to the use of private sector health care services. In the UK, some 22 per cent of subjects in the British Household Panel Survey (BHPS) reported some use of private health care in 1994–5, with use being quantitatively important for services where availability of NHS services is restricted or incomplete (Propper 2000). Such services include private dental care (used by about 13 per cent of the BHPS sample) and ophthalmic services (used by about 11 per cent of the BHPS sample). Public funding of access to nursing home care for older people is also severely restricted in England and Wales, although a less restrictive approach has recently been adopted in Scotland (Christie 2002). Much research interest has focused on the use of the private sector for elective hospital care because it is here that the NHS aims to provide universal access.

Just under 1 per cent of the BHPS sample reported using private inpatient services (Propper 2000). A survey of elective hospital treatments in 1997–8 found that some 14.5 per cent of elective hospital treatments were funded privately with about 10 per cent of these treatments being carried out in NHS hospitals (Williams *et al.* 2000). The source of funding was private health insurance for 81 per cent with payments from patients accounting for the remainder (Williams *et al.* 2000). The authors of the report observed that private health care was particularly heavily used for chronic conditions with serious health consequences for which there are long NHS waiting times. These included total hip replacement surgery (23 per cent privately funded, NHS waiting time 168 days), cataract extraction (17 per cent privately funded, NHS waiting time 144 days), and coronary artery bypass grafting (20 per cent privately funded, NHS waiting time 94 days). Private care was also used for procedures of uncertain effectiveness, such as operations for varicose veins, or for 'non-pathological' conditions, such as cosmetic surgery and gender reassignment which receive a low priority in the NHS.

The distribution of overall levels of utilisation of private elective hospital treatments has important implications for access to health care. In an ecological analysis, Williams and colleagues (Williams *et al.* 2001b) evaluated the distribution of private elective hospital treatment among eight English regions. They found that the proportion of private admissions ranged from 9 per cent in the Northern and Yorkshire region to 24 per cent in the North Thames region. Regions with more private hospital utilisation showed a lower proportion of the population reporting limiting long-term illness and a smaller number of NHS acute hospital beds, but a higher proportion of the population covered by private medical insurance. The authors concluded that at the regional level, NHS resources were distributed according to need, and that in more affluent but less needy areas, use of private services supplemented use of NHS services. However, they noted that within regions, differential use of NHS or private services could contribute to inequity. This observation was supported by Propper's analyses of individual-level data from the British Household Panel Survey sample (Propper 2000). Propper's results showed that, after controlling for health status, use of private care was strongly associated with higher household income, and with non-rented housing tenure. A particularly interesting feature of Propper's analyses was that not only did utilisation of private care contribute to inequity, but also users of private care were less likely to support the equity objectives of the NHS. People who used private care were more likely than users of NHS services to disagree with the statements that 'all health care should be free' or that it is 'unfair if money buys priority'.

Propper found that, from a longitudinal perspective, people often made use of either public and private sectors at different times (Propper 2000). The two sectors are also linked by the ability of medical staff to spend their spare time working in the private sector. It has been argued that the private sector will reduce demand on the National Health Service and thus increase access and quality for patients treated in the public sector. However, there may be incentives to medical staff to increase their efforts in the private sector and reduce their efforts in the public sector, with a consequent reduction in access. Iversen's theoretical work suggests that when consultant staff work in both sectors, there will be a tendency for waiting times to increase in the public sector (Iversen 1997).

In the UK, policy developments aimed at adjusting the balance between public and private health sectors have tended to be controversial because they address the ideological disagreements underlying health care provision. Examples include the use of private beds in NHS hospitals, the use of private finance in NHS capital projects, the use of tax relief to promote the uptake of private health insurance, proposed restrictions on the ability of NHS staff to work in the private sector, or the use of private capacity to treat patients on public sector waiting lists (Dean 2001). As well as being controversial, the consequences of these developments for access tend to be under-researched leading to a lack of evidence to inform policy.

Conclusions

The relevance of different financial barriers to health care is determined, to a large extent, by the predominant ideology influencing the development of a country's health system. In the US, where obtaining access to health care is viewed as the responsibility of the individual, personal financial barriers to access are arguably the more important. In the UK, where the health service aims to be more egalitarian, the state has taken responsibility for funding and providing health care. Here, the level of access achieved may be largely centrally determined. During the 1990s, market-style health sector reforms gave a greater role to incentives at the organisational level with the aim of achieving greater efficiency within health services. Achieving greater efficiency will often compromise equity objectives. This requires policy-makers to be more explicit about the specific objectives of organisations and systems, to monitor the levels of access achieved by different groups, and to design incentives and regulate providers in order to achieve the desired outcomes.

References

Benzeval, M. and Judge, K. (1996) 'Access to health care in England: continuing inequalities in the distribution of GPs', *Journal of Public Health Medicine*, 18: 33–40.

Bowling, A. (1996) 'Health care rationing: the public's debate', *British Medical Journal*, 312: 670–4.

Campbell, J.L., Ramsay, J. and Green, J. (2001) 'Practice size: impact on consultation length, workload and patient assessment of care', *British Journal of General Practice*, 51: 644–650.

Carroll, N.V. and Erwin, W.G. (1987) 'Patient shifting as a response to Medicare Prospective Payment', *Medical Care*, 25: 1161–7.

Christie, B. (2002) 'United Kingdom divided as Scotland introduces free personal care for elderly people', *British Medical Journal*, 324: 1542.

Culyer, A.J. (1989) 'Cost containment in Europe'. *Health Care Financing Review*, Annual supplement: 21–32.

Culyer, A.J., Brazier, J. and O'Donnell, O. (1988) 'Provider markets can potentially promote geographical equity since out of area purchases of services may release patients from dependence on locally acessibility of services'. Working paper No. 5. IHSM.

Dean, M. (2001) 'London – UK to embrace private-sector involvement in NHS?', *Lancet*, 358: 45.

Department of Health (2000) *The NHS Plan: A Plan for Investment, A Plan for Reform*. London: The Stationery Office.

Dixon, J., Harrison, A. and New, B. (1997) 'Funding in the NHS. Is the NHS underfunded?', *British Medical Journal*, 314: 58–61.

Donaldson, C. and Gerrard, K. (1989) 'Paying general practitioners: shedding light on the review of health services', *Journal of Royal College of General Practitioners*, 39: 114–17.

Donaldson, C. and Gerrard, K. (1992) *Economics of Health Care Financing: The Visible Hand*. Macmillan: Basingstoke.

Giuffrida, A., Gosden, T., Forland, F., Kristansen, I., Sergison, M., Leese, B., Pedersen, L. and Sutton, M. (2000) 'Target payments in primary care: effects on professional practice and health care outcomes (Cochrane Review)'. In *The Cochrane Library*, 4. Oxford: Update Software.

Glied, S. (1998) 'Getting the incentives right for children', *Health Services Research*, 33: 1143–60.

Gosden, T., Forland, F., and Kristiansen, I., Sutton, M. Leese, B., Giuffrida, A., Sergison, M. and Pedersen, L. (2000) 'Capitation, salary, fee-for-service and mixed systems of payment: effect on the behaviour of primary care physicians (Cochrane Review)'. In *The Cochrane Library*, 3. Oxford: Update Software.

Gosden, T., Williams, J., Petchey, R., Leese, B. and Sibbald, B. (2002) 'Salaried contracts in UK general practice: a study of job satisfaction and stress', *Journal of Health Services Research Policy*, 7: 26–33.

Gravelle, H. and Sutton, M. (1998) 'Trends in geographical inequalities in provision of general practitioners in England and Wales', *Lancet*, 352: 1910.

Gravelle, H. and Sutton, M. (2001) 'Inequality in the geographical distribution of general practitioners in England and Wales 1974–1995', *Journal of Health Services Research Policy*, 6: 6–13.

Haber, S.G. and Mitchell, J.B. (1999) 'Access to physicians' services for vulnerable Medicare beneficiaries', *Inquiry – The Journal of Health Care Organization Provision and Financing*, 36: 445–60.

Hadorn, D.C. and Brook, R.H. (1991) 'The health care resource allocation debate – defining our terms', *Journal of American Medical Association*, 266: 3328–31.

Hamilton, V. (1993) 'The Medicare hospice benefit – the effectiveness of price incentives in health-care', *Journal of Economics*, 24: 605–24.

Hannay, D.R., Usherwood, T.P. and Platts, M. (1992) 'Practice organization before and after the new contract: a survey of general practices in Sheffield', *British Journal of General Practice*, 42: 517–20.

Horder, J., Bosanquet, N. and Stocking, B. (1986) 'Ways of influencing the behaviour of general practitioners', *Journal of the Royal College of General Practitioners*, 36: 517–21.

Hughes, D. and McGuire, A. (1995) 'Patient charges and the utilisation of NHS prescription medicines: some estimates using a cointegration procedure', *Health Economics*, 4: 213–20.

Hughes, D. and Yule, B. (1991) 'Incentives and the remuneration of general practitioners', HERU Discussion Paper, University of Aberdeen.

Hughes, D. and Yule, B. (1992) 'The effect of per-item fees on the behaviour of general practitioners', *Journal of Health Economics*, 11: 413–37.

Iversen, T. (1997) 'The effect of a private sector on the waiting time in a national health service', *Journal of Health Economics*, 16: 381–96.

Krasnik, A., Groenewegen, P., Pedersen, P., Scholten, P.V., Mooney, G., Gottshau, A., Flierman, H. and Damsgard, M. (1990) 'Changing remuneration systems: effects on activity in general practice', *British Medical Journal*, 300: 1698–701.

Lu, M.S. and Donaldson, C. (2000) 'Performance-based contracts and provider efficiency –the state of the art', *Disease Management and Health Outcomes*, 7: 127–37.

Lundberg, L., Johannesson, M., Dag, I. and Borgquist, L. (1998) 'Effects of user charges on the use of prescription medicines in different socioeconomic groups', *Health Policy*, 44: 123–34.

Mayer, M.L., Stearns, S.C., Norton, E.C. and Rozier, R.G. (2000) 'The effects of Medicaid expansions and reimbursement increases on dentists' participation', *Inquiry – The Journal of Health Care Organization Provision and Financing*, 37: 33–44.

Mufti, M.H. (2000) 'A case for user charges in hospitals', *Saudi Medical Journal*, 21: 5–7.

New, B. (1996) 'The rationing agenda in the NHS', *British Medical Journal*, 312: 1593–601.

Newhouse, J. (1996) *Free for all?: Lessons from the Rand Health Insurance Experiment.* Cambridge, MA: Harvard University Press.

Pande, P.N. (1998) 'Time for reflection after the Bristol case', *Lancet*, 352: 232–3.

Parmanum, J., Field, D., Rennie, J. and Steer, P. (2000) 'National census of availability of neonatal intensive care. British Association for Perinatal Medicine', *British Medical Journal*, 321: 727–9.

Propper, C. (2000) 'The demand for private health care in the UK', *Journal of Health Economics*, 19: 855–76.

Quinn, M.J., Martinez-Garcia, C. and Berrino, F. (1998) 'Variations in survival from breast cancer in Europe by age and country, 1978–1989', *European Journal of Cancer*, 34: 2204–11.

Rice, T.H. (1983) 'The impact of changing Medicare reimbursement rates on physician induced demand', *Medical Care*, 21: 803–15.

Rice, T. and Morrison, K. (1994) 'Patient cost sharing for medical services: A review of the literature and implications for health care reform', *Medical Care Review*, 51: 235–87.

Rosko, M.D. and Broyles, R.W. (1987) 'Short-term responses of hospitals to the DRG prospective pricing mechanism in New Jersey', *Medical Care*, 25: 88–99.

Saltman, R.B. (2002) 'Regulating incentives: the past and present role of the state in health care systems', *Social Science and Medicine*, 54: 1677–84.

Sassi, F., Archard, L. and Le Grand, J. (2001) 'Equity and the economic evaluation of health care', *Health Technology Assessment*, 5(3): i–138.

Scheffler, R.M., Foreman, S.E., Feldstein, P.J. and Hu, T.W. (1996) 'A multi-equation model of payments and public access to services: the case of dentistry', *Applied Economics*, 28: 1359–68.

Stoelwinder, J.U. (1994) 'Casemix payment in the real world of running a hospital', *Medical Journal of Australia*, 161: S15–S18.

Tobias, J.S. (1988) 'What went wrong at Exeter?', *British Medical Journal*, 297: 372–3.

Travis, K.M. (1999) 'Physician payment and prenatal care access for heterogeneous patients', *Economic Inquiry*, 37: 86–102.

Wagstaff, A. and van Doorslaer, E. (1992) 'Equity in the finance of health care: some international comparisons', *Journal of Health Economics*, 11: 361–87.

Wagstaff, A., van Doorslaer, E., van der Burg, H., Calonge, S., Christiansen, T., Citoni, G., Gerdtham, U.G., Gerfin, M., Gross, L., Hakinnen, U., Johnson, P., John, J., Klavus, J., Lachaud, C., Lauritsen, J., Leu, R., Nolan, B., Peran, E., Pereira, J., Propper, C., Puffer, F., Rochaix, L., Rodriguez, M., Schellhorn, M. and Winkelhake, O. (1999) 'Equity in the finance of health care: some further international comparisons', *Journal of Health Economics*, 18: 263–90.

Wanless, D. (2001) *Securing Our Future Health: Taking a Long Term View*. London: Her Majesty's Treasury.

Wanless, D. (2002) *Securing Our Future Health: Taking a Long Term View. Final Report.* London: Her Majesty's Treasury.

Williams, B., Whatmough, P., McGill, J. and Rushton, L. (2000) 'Private funding of elective hospital treatment in England and Wales, 1997–8: national survey', *British Medical Journal*, 320: 904–5.

Williams, J., Petchey, R., Gosden, T., Leese, B. and Sibbald, B. (2001a) 'A profile of PMS salaried GP contracts and their impact on recruitment', *Family Practice*, 18: 283–7.

Williams, B., Whatmough, P., McGill, J. and Rushton, L. (2001b) 'Impact of private funding on access to elective hospital treatment in the regions of England and Wales – National records survey', *European Journal of Public Health*, 11: 402–6.

Chapter 7

Access to health care in the United States

Sarah C. Blake, Kenneth E. Thorpe and Kelly G. Howell

Introduction

In the United States, there is no national health care service. The ability of Americans to gain access to health care is not simplified through any systematic approach. Instead, there is an inconsistent array of private and public programmes that offer health care to some but not all in the US, indicating an uneven and evolving approach to the provision and financing of health care. There have been a number of attempts to achieve a universal system of care, most notably the Clinton administration's Health Security Act in the early 1990s, but the provision of comprehensive and affordable health care services is still not guaranteed to all Americans (Starr 1992; Derickson 2002; Iglehart 1992). Ongoing ideological debate about this issue centres around whether health care in America is a fundamental right or a luxury. This discussion is complicated by the very complex and rapidly changing organisation and management of health care in the United States. As a result of the changing structure of the American health care delivery system, together with the increasing influence of the health care system on the US economy and on the health status of millions of Americans, access to health care has become an enormous challenge to policymakers, health care providers, and consumers.

The availability, utilisation, and financing of health care is influenced by a range of stakeholders in the US health care system which includes the government, employers, providers, and insurers or health plans. Understanding the roles of these players and the enormous variability in their responsibilities and abilities to provide health care helps to shed light on the growing concern over access to health care in America. We will also examine some of the many factors that influence the accessibility of health care for consumers in America, including differences in personal income, employment, health care coverage, geography, health insurance, and stark economic and social differences among its culturally diverse population.

Availability of providers

In order to understand how or why a population has access to health care, we must first examine the supply and availability of health care services. We begin with a brief discussion of the characteristics of the US delivery system and how changes in this system lead to differences in the potential to gain access to health care.

Health services in America are provided through a loosely structured delivery system of public and private providers, organised primarily at the local level (DeLew *et al.* 1992). Providers in this delivery system include physicians, hospitals, community health centres, public health departments and other specialty health care clinics. Community hospitals comprise the largest proportion of hospitals in the US. Of almost 6,000 hospitals reported in 1999, just under 5,000 were community-based hospitals, while 264 were federal hospitals and 670 were non-federal, non-community hospitals. Community hospitals are more likely to be located in urban rather than rural locations (see Box 7.1). American Hospital Association (AHA) data reveal that in 1999, there were 2,767 urban community hospitals versus 2,189 rural community hospitals (American Hospital Association 2001).

Physicians are likely to be either in solo practice or part of an organised, coordinated care system, such as managed care, and in suburban or urban locations. Community health centres and other public health clinics are government-funded institutions and are located in urban or rural areas. These sites are staffed by physicians as well as allied health professionals, such as nurses and physician assistants, and most commonly serve as safety nets for patients who are not covered by insurance, who cannot afford to pay for health care services, and who do not have a regular source of care (National Association of Community Health Centers 2002).

As Aday and colleagues indicate, the major policy concerns regarding the availability of these providers have shifted from the issue of supply to that of distribution (Aday *et al.* 1993). Over the past 30 years, increased training of medical personnel and new hospital construction led to an overall increase in the number of providers and facilities. The number of active physicians per 100,000 population increased 67.1 per cent from 1970 to 1996 (Health Services Resources and Services Administration 2000). The number of hospital beds per 1,000 population expanded by over a third from 1940 to 1980, though recent estimates indicate this number has declined slightly in recent years (National Center for Health Statistics 1990; National Center for Health Statistics 2001; Aday *et al.* 1993). This growth, however, has occurred in mostly suburban locations. Despite general increases in the physician-to-population ratio, rural and urban underserved communities are confronted with problems of geographic maldistribution. Rural hospital closures, financially stressed urban hospitals, and provider flight from or reluctance to locate in these same areas have contributed to this problem as well as to an insufficient supply of services to these communities (Council on Graduate Medical Education 1998; Aday *et al.* 1993; Hicks and Glen 1991).

The types of health care services, and the extent to which services are available, vary greatly among these providers. Community hospitals, the most common type of US hospitals, tend to be short-term hospitals offering a range of general health services as well as special hospital services, such as obstetrics and gynaecology,

Box 7.1 Glossary of terms

Urban/suburban/rural: The terms 'urban', 'suburban' and 'rural' are general descriptors used to indicate geographical designations. A rural hospital, for instance, would be located outside a metropolitan statistical area (MSA), which is a geographically defined, integrated social and economic unit with a large population nucleus. An urban hospital is located within a metropolitan statistical area, usually within or close to a major city with a large population. A suburban hospital may be located in an MSA but usually with a smaller population and not located centrally in a major city.

Community hospitals: Community hospitals are all non-federal, short-term, general and special hospitals whose facilities and services are available to the public.

Public health clinics: Public health clinics are typically not-for-profit health clinics, run by governmental and non-governmental entities, providing primary health care services to the public at little or no cost. Such clinics may be stand-alone clinics or located within organised entities, such as community health centres or public health departments.

Underserved communities: Underserved communities include population groups that have economic barriers or cultural and/or linguistic access barriers to primary medical care services. Approximately 53 million people in the United States live in medically underserved communities.

Non-physicians: Non-physicians include all allied health personnel, including nurses, physician assistants, physical therapists, occupational therapists, as well as dentists, dental assistants, and mental health professionals.

Managed care: Managed care is a health care plan that integrates the financing and delivery of health services by using arrangements with selected health care providers to provide services for covered individuals. Plans are generally financed using capitation fees. There are significant financial incentives for members of the plan to use the health care providers associated with the plan. The plan includes formal programmes for quality assurance and utilisation review.

Point-of-service (POS) plans: A type of managed care plan, POS plan participants usually choose a Primary Care Physician (PCP) from those participating in the plan's provider network. Care received in-network under the direction of the PCP is typically provided at maximum benefits. A POS plan participant also has the option to go out-of-network for eligible services and receive reduced benefits with deductibles and coinsurance.

Sources: American Hospital Association (2001);
Centers for Disease Control and Prevention (2001);
United States Department of Health and Human Services (2002).

eye, ear, nose, and throat services, rehabilitation, and orthopaedic services. Federal hospitals offer a wide variety of health services but these are only available to specific populations, including military personnel, veterans, or Native Americans (part of the government sponsored Indian Health Service) (Centers for Disease Control 2001). Non-federal, non-community hospitals include those for mental health, tuberculosis and other respiratory diseases and include both long-term and short-term hospitals (Centers for Disease Control 2001). While there are both private and public hospitals, public hospitals that receive federal financing have an obligation to accept poor and medically indigent patients. According to the American Hospital Association, 16 per cent of this medically underserved population considers the hospital emergency department as their usual source of care. Having no regular source of care and little ability to pay for care, many uninsured persons rely on public hospital emergency rooms for basic health care services, as well as enabling services such as counselling and social services (DeLew et al. 1992; American Hospital Association 2000).

Public hospitals are just one of the many types of safety net providers that provide basic primary care services to the poor and uninsured in America. Located in primarily rural and urban locations, safety net providers have received much attention in recent years because of the increasing role they play in providing access to care and the growing financial crises these providers now face (McAlearney 2002; Asplin 2001; Institute of Medicine 2000). The safety net is a health care system in its own right. It comprises doctors, nurses, and others who work in public hospitals, non-profit community hospitals, community-based and school-based health centres, as well as public health clinics, and to some degree private practices. Because these safety net providers are financed with public funds, they have a legal obligation to provide health care services for free, or for a nominal fee, to anyone who seeks care. The Bureau of Primary Health Care, a federal health care agency within the US Department of Health and Human Services, administers several programmes that provide grant funding to these safety net providers, including the Community and Migrant Health Center Program and the Health Care for the Homeless Program. Other government funding goes toward specific health care services for the underserved, including family planning, HIV/AIDs, and maternal and child health care (National Governers Association 2000).

Trends towards increased specialisation of health professionals also affect the availability of health care in America. The health professions workforce in the US is characterised by an oversupply of specialists and an undersupply of generalists or primary care physicians who are willing to practice in rural and/or underserved areas. The literature suggests that strong market forces, and increased attention paid by medical schools to specialty care curricula, have influenced health professionals' practice choices (Council on Graduate Medical Education 1998; Iglehart 1993; Rosenblatt and Lishner 1991; Lee 1991). As a result, there is a significant lack of primary care services available for medically underserved communities, especially rural communities (Politzer et al. 1991; Hicks and Glen 1991). Though there may be greater willingness by non-physicians to work in these underserved areas, the availability of certain health services, such as specialised health care and dental care, remains a significant problem because of the lack of providers as well as lack of health care coverage for these services (Hart 1997; Bureau of Health Professions 1993).

Over the past few decades, federal and state initiatives have tried to address the access problems related to the shortage of health professionals in rural and urban underserved areas, also referred to as Health Professional Shortage Areas (HPSAs). Scholarships and educational debt forgiveness programmes have been offered for years through the National Health Service Corps and Indian Health Service for health professionals who agree to serve in these areas (Cullen *et al.* 1997; Politzer *et al.* 1991). In addition, incentives have been used to recruit international medical graduates to serve in Health Professional Shortage Areas and other underserved locales. Typically, these graduates are offered waivers of the foreign residence requirement, or what are know as J-1 visas, in exchange for the health professional's agreement to serve in a rural underserved community (Orloff and Tymann 1995).

Availability of health insurance

The accessibility of health care services depends on the availability and type of health care insurance coverage. Approximately 64.1 per cent of Americans have private health insurance, mostly provided through employer-sponsored plans (Current Population Survey 2001). People without access to employer-sponsored insurance can access health insurance in their own right, usually through the individual health insurance market (Claxton 2002). For reasons explained in greater detail below, employers are concerned with containing costs and have contracted increasingly with health plans that offer managed care arrangements. The net effect of increased managed care has been stricter control on the availability of health services for enrollees, and financial incentives to physicians and hospitals aimed at cutting both services and costs (Kuttner 1999). Furthermore, managed care products, like health maintenance organisations (HMOs) or point-of-service plans, often vary greatly in the health benefit packages and network of providers offered to enrollees (Rosenbaum *et al.* 2002; Bodenheimer 1992).

Public health insurance programmes cover approximately 24.2 per cent of the US population (Current Population Survey 2001). The Medicare programme is a federal health insurance programme that covers individuals aged 65 years and older who have worked for at least ten years in the workforce or who are disabled. Medicare was established in 1965 primarily as a programme to ensure access to care for elderly persons; it now covers over 39 million Americans (Center for Medicare and Medicaid Services 2002; Wilensky 1995). It is structured in two parts: Part A covers all inpatient hospital services and is automatically available for eligible persons; Part B is a supplemental programme, purchased individually by beneficiaries, and is financed by general revenues of the federal government and in part by premium payments from the elderly. Part B coverage pays for doctors' services, outpatient hospital services, and other services not typically covered under Part A, such as physical therapy and home health care.

Medicare has traditionally been considered a success story, partly because of the freedom beneficiaries have in provider choice, and the minimal cost-sharing involved (Wilensky 1995). In recent years, concerns have grown over the financial stability of the Medicare programme and enrollees' access to certain services, especially prescription drugs (Kaiser Commission Medicaid and the Uninsured 2001d; Wilensky 2001). While a very limited number of prescription drugs are available through Medicare, there are several legislative proposals currently under debate to incorporate the coverage of outpatient prescription drugs into Medicare Part B. This debate over a Medicare prescription drug benefit centres on several unresolved issues, such as the cost to the federal government, the cost to individual Medicare beneficiaries, and the impact on the private insurance industry (Dewar and Goldstein 2002).

The Medicaid programme is an assistance programme for over 40 million low-income pregnant women and children, elderly, and disabled persons funded by federal, state, and local taxes. Each state administers its own Medicaid programme within minimum federal guidelines. Most states have great flexibility in setting their own eligibility guidelines and health benefit packages but some services, such as family planning services and childhood immunisations, are mandated by the federal government and must be available to all enrollees. In recent years, many state Medicaid programmes have begun to institute managed care, changing from a fee-for-service system, and offering or mandating their beneficiaries to enrol in managed care plans. Citing concerns over rising costs, states' decision to move towards managed care has also limited the ability of enrollees to access care (Waitzman et al. 2002; Iglehart 1995). Recent health plan withdrawal from Medicaid managed-care programmes and provider reluctance to accept new Medicaid enrollees has contributed to the overall lack of availability for this population (Mirvis et al. 2002; Kaiser Commission on Medicaid and the Uninsured 2001c; Felt-Lisk et al. 2001).

The most recent public health insurance programme is the State Children's Health Insurance Program (SCHIP), which was created in 1997. SCHIP is also a federal-state programme that is administered by each state. SCHIP covers low-income uninsured children and is increasingly being expanded by states to cover parents of SCHIP children who do not qualify for Medicaid.

Those with no health insurance, approximately 16 per cent of the non-elderly US population, are forced to rely on public health departments, community health clinics, or public hospitals for health care services. With the exception of some specialty health clinics that provide specific health services, such as HIV/AIDs and family planning services, uninsured persons have access only to very basic primary care services through these public providers. Preventive health care services are rarely available and most uninsured do not have access to care for more serious and chronic conditions (American College of Physicians 2000; Bindman et al. 1996; Hafner-Eaton 1993).

Lack of health insurance

Numerous studies of access in the US have demonstrated that health insurance coverage is an important predictor of the utilisation of health care services (Strunk and Cunningham 2002; American College of Physicians 2000; Cunningham and Kemper 1998; Aday *et al.* 1993) and the greatest personal barrier to health care in America is the lack of health insurance. Over 40 million Americans were uninsured in 2001. Despite the economic growth and low unemployment rates in recent years, the number of uninsured in the US is expected to remain steady if not increase (Holahan 2002; Hoffman and Pohl 2002; Kaiser Commission on Medicaid and the Uninsured 2003).

The uninsured face great financial difficulties in paying for their health care and thus rely on the health care safety net and other charitable sources of care (Holahan 2002; Cunningham and Kemper 1998; Lipson and Naierman 1996). Because of the great variability in the safety net services available in US communities, significant gaps exist in the use of these health care services for the uninsured. The uninsured are less likely to have a regular source of care or to have seen a physician within the previous year (Holahan 2002; Kaiser Commission on Medicaid and the Uninsured 2002a). For instance, uninsured children are 70 per cent less likely than insured children to have received medical care for common conditions such as ear infections. Both uninsured adults and children are less likely to receive preventive care. In addition, the uninsured are more likely than those with insurance to be hospitalised for conditions that could have been avoided, such as pneumonia and uncontrolled diabetes, and to be treated at later stages of disease because of a delay in seeking care (Kaiser Commission on Medicaid and the Uninsured 2003; Bradley *et al.* 2002; Government Accounting Office 2001b; Pappas *et al.* 1997; Ayanian *et al.* 1993).

Income and employment status are two major determinants of health care insurance. As noted previously, there are varied sources of health insurance, including private insurance, Medicare, Medicaid, SCHIP, even military health insurance for veterans and their families. In order to be eligible for private insurance, individuals must be offered and accept health insurance through an employer, or a family member's employer. Studies show that many working families are uninsured either because they cannot afford the cost-sharing requirements of private insurance or because their employers have not offered this type of employment benefit (Rowland 2002; American College of Physicians 2000; Government Accounting Office 1997). Out-of-pocket payments for private insurance, including premiums, deductibles, or co-payments, have risen at a faster rate than overall health expenditures in the US (Kuttner 1999). Recent figures indicate that nearly 30 per cent of workers in small businesses have no health coverage. Uninsured rates are particularly high among those who work full-time but only for part of a year (such as laid-off or temporary employees) (Hoffman and Pohl 2002; Government Accounting Office 2001b; American College of Physicians 2000).

Only people with little or no income are eligible for public health insurance. Medicaid and SCHIP help fill in the gaps in insurance for some of the lowest income people, but these programmes are directed primarily at low-income children, the disabled, and pregnant women. Low-income childless adults and parents are less likely to be covered through these programmes and these programmes' eligibility criteria vary across the United States. The reality is that low-income individuals have a high chance of being uninsured. Nearly 64 per cent of the uninsured come from low-income families earning less than 200 per cent of the federal poverty level (an income of $27,476 for a family of three) (Rowland 2002). Low-income uninsured people face serious problems obtaining health care with 16.4 per cent reporting an unmet need in 2001 (Strunk and Cunningham 2002).

Financial barriers to utilisation

There are two other types of financial barriers that influence access to health care in the United States. Personal financing issues, such as income and the ability to pay for health-related costs, are one such type of barrier. As discussed above, insurance and employment as well as income can affect individuals' utilisation of services. The second type of barrier includes the fiscal constraints inherent in the health care system. With health care spending at an all-time high and a weakened economy, the government as well as the private health care sector are faced with budget constraints and other financial pressures that may lead to further deterioration in access to care (Strunk and Cunningham 2002; Marks 2002; Miller 2001). Health care costs have been cited as the greatest personal financial barrier to getting needed care (Rowland 2002; Strunk and Cunningham 2002; Government Accounting Office 1998). Among people with an unmet need or who delayed care, more than 60 per cent reported difficulty getting care because of worries about costs. Cost was overwhelmingly the main barrier to care for the uninsured, with over 93 per cent of the uninsured citing cost as the reason for difficulty in getting care in 2001. Even those people with insurance cited cost as a barrier (Strunk and Cunningham 2002).

The affordability of health care has become an issue for all Americans. Out-of-pocket spending, which includes expenditures for coinsurance and deductibles required by insurers, as well as direct payments for services not covered by a third party, amounted to $188.8 billion in 1997, or 17.2 per cent of all national health expenditures (Iglehart 1999). For persons with health insurance through their employer or as a dependent of an employee, annual contributions to this coverage averaged around $2,000 for individuals, and $6,000 for families in 1997, declining slightly in 2001 (Rowland 2002; Levitt and Lundy 1998).

Health care costs for the uninsured and people with low incomes are also great barriers to care. Cost-sharing requirements of public health programmes, such as Medicaid and Medicare, have placed great financial burdens on these populations. In addition, reports indicate that recently unemployed persons are not able to take advantage of the option to continue their previous health insurance by purchasing temporary coverage because of high premium costs. This safety net coverage requires laid-off workers to pay 102 per cent of the premium costs. Given the loss of employment and loss of income, this is particularly difficult for individuals who had been low-paid workers (Schoen 2001; Kaiser Commission Medicaid and the Uninsured 2001a; Lambrew 2001). Adding to this problem, approximately 725,000 workers who have lost their jobs since the start of the most recent US economic recession have also lost their health insurance (Families USA 2001).

High health care costs are an urgent problem for both the public and private health care sectors. In 1990, 33 per cent of US health care expenditures were from public sources, including 18 per cent from the federal government and 15 per cent from state and local governments, while 29 per cent were from private businesses, 35 per cent were from individuals, and 3 per cent were from non-patient revenues (philanthropic funds, providers' interest income, etc.) (Aday et al. 1993). Federal government expenditures for health care costs through public programmes such as Medicaid and Medicare are well over $300 billion and are expected to grow at an annual rate of 8 per cent over the next ten years (Smith 2002; Congressional Budget Office 1997). The Medicaid programme, in particular, is causing great financial stress for states, accounting now for approximately 20 per cent of state spending (National Governors Association 2002). The private sector, which assumes a large role in financial health care through employer-based coverage, is currently experiencing a dramatic slowdown in health insurance spending. While the annual growth rate of private health insurance expenditures increased from 17 per cent in 1965 to 27 per cent in 1980, the annual growth rate of private health expenditures has dropped dramatically to less than 3 per cent in 1994 and 1995 (Aday et al. 1993; Congressional Budget Office 1997).

The financial stress faced by the public and private health care systems has led to reform efforts that aim to reduce health care costs. Such reform efforts have included imposing stricter insurance eligibility criteria, reduced health benefit coverage, increased patient cost-sharing measures, and restricted rates of reimbursement to health care providers (Iglehart 1999; Aday et al. 1993). As a result, individuals are less likely to be covered, to have access to comprehensive health services, and to be able to pay for health care. Physicians and other providers are in constant conflict with health insurers over decreasing expenditures and decreasing attention given to quality of care (Sultz and Young 1997).

Organisational barriers to access

As in the UK, there are many organisational barriers to accessing health care in the United States. Such barriers exist primarily because of the great variation in the service configuration of the public and private health care systems. Provider ratios, provider network standards, and specialty care referral arrangements, for instance, differ greatly among health plans and across state public health care programmes (Rosenbaum et al. 2002). Patients' ability to navigate through these systems may be affected by the location of providers, available transportation, linguistically appropriate health care materials and bilingual staff, accommodations for the disabled, as well as availability of appointments (Strunk and Cunningham 2002). These barriers represent physical, geographic, and social system limitations that are shaped by the organisation of health care in the United States.

Efforts to eliminate these types of organisational barriers have focused on strengthening the infrastructure of the US health care system. This includes adding primary care as well as specialty care providers to rural and medically underserved locations, providing more interpreters at hospitals and other safety net locations, and arranging for transportation services for those in need (Fehr-Synder 2002; Fiscella *et al.* 2002; National Rural Health Association 1999; McKinney 1998; Guidry *et al.* 1997). In addition, research indicates that eliminating certain barriers such as long waiting times for appointments and improving the cultural competency or sensitivity of providers will increase patients' use of health care services (Mofidi *et al.* 2002; Office of Minority Health 2001; Cunningham *et al.* 1999; Flores *et al.* 1998; Flores 2000).

There are a number of different approaches taken in the United State to evaluate the relevance or effectiveness of access to health care. These evaluations may be made on national as well as state levels. They may seek to evaluate health care programmes, health care plans, or the experiences of health care consumers and their ability to access basic health services. Evaluations may be undertaken by federal and/or state agencies, private health plans, academic research institutions, or private research firms. In addition, depending on the specific measure of access, evaluations may use qualitative or quantitative methodologies.

Standards for the provision and delivery of health care have been developed and these include widely accepted measures of access which health plans and providers are required to adhere to. Examples include the requirements that providers are located within a certain distance, that appointments must be available within certain timeframes, that health care facilities meet requirements of the Americans With Disabilities Act (ADA), or that translation services or bilingual health care materials are available to patients. One study of Medicaid managed care contracts found that although most health plans incorporated such access standards and required at least some type of standard, the variability in these service configurations among states might have differing impacts on patients' ability to access some health care services. For prenatal visits, for example, California requires a first-time appointment be made within one week, while the District of Columbia allows up to 20 days for a woman's first prenatal visit to be scheduled. In West Virginia, beneficiaries are only required to travel up to 35 miles to access a specialty care provider, while in Texas, a beneficiary may have to travel up to 75 miles to access a specialty care provider (Rosenbaum *et al.* 2002). This difference may reflect the states' geography, but it also may reflect the differences in service delivery systems and potential access barriers.

Equity and access

The inherent goal of an equitable health care system is to provide 'the freedom and equality of opportunity to obtain adequate and effective medical care' (Aday *et al.* 1993: 126). Equity concerns the notion of providing equal access to health care resources to meet the needs of all groups of people (see Chapter 3). In the United States, this is a particularly difficult challenge because of the wide variation in the organisation and delivery of health care across the states and in the health needs of many different groups of people. The diverse strategies employed across the states to meet those needs has resulted in different public and private health care programmes that offer different levels of health care coverage and benefits, and various mechanisms to finance services. Consequently, great inequities exist in accessing health care in the United States.

Inequity in access to health care is a strong determinant of health outcomes. Populations that experience some inequality or inequity in access to health care also tend to have poorer health outcomes. In the US, this is particularly true for low-income uninsured and minority populations. For example, low-income populations, especially poor children, tend to have worse oral health and make fewer dental visits because of a lack of dental care coverage and availability of dental health care providers (Mouradian *et al.* 2000; Mueller *et al.* 1998). Low-income and minority women tend to have higher breast cancer mortality rates and lower survival rates because of the lack of access and delayed screening (American Cancer Society 2002; Bradley *et al.* 2002; Boyer-Chammard *et al.* 1999). Data from the National Cancer Institute show that the five-year survival rate for breast cancer is 72.5 per cent for black women, versus 87.6 per cent for white women (Ries *et al.* 2002). Inadequate access to affordable treatment and health coverage for HIV/AIDs services are reasons more low-income and minority populations are dying faster from the disease (Herbert 2001; Center for Disease Control 2000).

Three recent reports on the uninsured demonstrate the serious consequences of the lack of health care coverage. Findings from an Institute of Medicine study indicate that Americans without health insurance are more likely to have poorer health and die prematurely than those with insurance. Uninsured patients with colon or breast cancer face up to a 50 per cent greater chance of dying than patients with private coverage. Uninsured victims of trauma also are more likely to die from their injuries (Institute of Medicine 2002b). Even being uninsured for just one year seems to affect a person's perceived health status. A study recently released by Ayanian *et al.* (2000) indicates that even short-term uninsured adults (those uninsured for a year or less) report worse health outcomes than insured adults. Based on the Behavioral Risk Factor Surveillance System, a survey of more than 100,000 US adults, findings indicate that short-term uninsured adults were more likely to have unmet health needs and to report their health status as fair or poor (Ayanian *et al.* 2000).

An extensive review of the health services research literature by researchers from the Urban Institute (Hadley 2002), a highly respected American research organisation, indicates that uninsured persons have worse health outcomes, especially poorer birth outcomes, than the insured. Research has demonstrated that having health insurance increases timely initiation of prenatal care, promotes access to caesarian-section deliveries for high-risk births, and increases access to neonatal intensive care for high-risk babies. General health outcomes also tend to be worse for the uninsured. Those with no health insurance are 50 per cent less likely than insured persons to use medical care, and they also have a 5 to 15 per cent higher mortality rate (Hadley 2002).

Much of the literature on equity and access relates to socioeconomic disparities in health care. Ethnic disparities in health care are also important. The Institute of Medicine (2002b) recently released a study that presents compelling evidence that ethnic minorities receive lower-quality health care than whites, even after controlling for health insurance, income, age, and severity of condition. Minorities are less likely to be given appropriate cardiac medications, such as beta blockers or thrombolytic drugs, and are less likely to receive kidney dialysis or transplants. In one study of dialysis patients, 30 per cent of the white patients were put on a transplant list, while only 13.5 per cent of the African American patients were put on a transplant list (Institute of Medicine 2002a). Ethnic minorities are more likely to be diagnosed with cancer at advanced stages, to be diagnosed with a psychiatric disorder, and to be hospitalised for pregnancy-related complications. They are less likely to be screened for certain types of cancer and less likely to receive prenatal care (Institute of Medicine 2002a; Schneider *et al.* 2002). African Americans are 32–70 per cent less likely to receive bypass surgery than whites and 13–40 per cent less likely to receive coronary angioplasty. African Americans are also 41–73 per cent less likely than whites to receive sophisticated treatments for HIV, such as antiviral therapies. African Americans and Asian Americans are more than six times as likely as whites to be diagnosed with alcohol or substance abuse problems (Morehouse Medical Effectiveness Treatment Center 1999). Other work supporting these findings also indicates that minorities experience more communication problems and have an inconsistent relationship with their physicians, because of language barriers and a lack of doctors in minority communities (Fehr-Synder 2002; Collins *et al.* 2001; Morehouse Medical Effectiveness Treatment Center 1999).

Immigrants' access to health care has been affected by recent public policy changes. The Personal Responsibility and Work Opportunity Act of 1996 (PRWORA) instituted a fundamental change to the US welfare system by banning most forms of public assistance and social services for legal and non-legal immigrants who have not become citizens. In particular, PRWORA restricted Medicaid eligibility of immigrants and effectively denied access to most health care services (except emergency services) previously afforded to them (Weitzman 1997; Ku and Matani 2001; Maloy *et al.* 2000). This has become a significant problem, since most immigrants are low-income and uninsured and had relied on Medicaid for health care coverage. Research has indicated that immigrants are experiencing greater inequities in ambulatory care, primary care, and mental health, as well as worse health outcomes as a result (Kaiser Commission on Medicaid and the Uninsured 2001e; Ku and Matani 2001; Hudman 2000; Maloy *et al.* 2000).

Gender differences also exist in health care access. A lack of affordable and adequate health care coverage remains the greatest barrier to access for American women. Almost 6 million women lack health care insurance in the United States and since welfare reform this rate of uninsurance has grown by half (Guyer *et al.* 2002; Mann *et al.* 2002). Uninsured and low-income women are less likely to obtain needed care, specifically preventive care, than those with insurance (Kaiser Family Foundation 2002; Lambrew 2001; Collins *et al.* 1999). Even for insured women, access to certain health care services remains difficult. Some family planning services, such as certain contraceptives, infertility treatments, and sterilisation services, are excluded from most health insurance plans. Long-term care, as another example, remains a problem for women, who constitute a majority of long-term care recipients, because Medicare does not cover long-term services (National Women Law Center 2001).

Policy responses

Recent efforts to reduce disparities in health care access have focused mainly on the expansion of health care coverage. In the past decade, universal health care coverage was proposed by the Clinton administration. This would have extended health insurance coverage to all Americans, either through a private or public health plan. In addition to universal coverage, the Clinton plan would have changed how Americans choose their plans. Today, most Americans receive their health insurance through their employer. For the most part, employers select the plans, and employees select based on these limited choices. The Clinton proposal would have redirected this function from the employer to large purchasing pools. This would not only have changed who sponsored the plans, but would have expanded dramatically the number of plans employees and others would select. The redistributive components of the Clinton proposal attracted opposition from some employers and private health plans, contributing to its demise.

Other efforts have included the use of federal Medicaid waivers, such as Section 1115 waivers, which allow states to expand Medicaid eligibility for families and children. Within the past two years, the Bush administration created the Health Insurance Flexibility and Accountability Initiative, which allows states to expand Medicaid coverage to parents and other adults of Medicaid-eligible children.

Interest in expanding health care coverage to low-income children led to the enactment of SCHIP in 1997. The programme targets uninsured children under 19 with family incomes below 200 per cent of the federal poverty level (FPL) who are not eligible for Medicaid or covered by private insurance. SCHIP is a federal-state matching block grant programme, with $40 billion in federal funds allocated to this programme over ten years. As of June 2000, over 2 million children in all 50 states were enrolled in SCHIP (Kaiser Commission on Medicaid and the Uninsured 2001b).

Finally, recent efforts to address health care disparities have focused on expanding specific types of health care services, including breast and cervical cancer treatment, treatment for Alzheimer's, and access to prescription drugs. In October of 2000, the Breast and Cervical Cancer Prevention and Treatment Act (BCCPTA) was passed by Congress to allow states the option of expanding Medicaid to low-income women diagnosed with breast and/or cervical cancer. Before this time, low-income uninsured women with breast and cervical cancer had to rely on charity care for treatment. The Breast and Cervical Cancer Prevention and Treatment Act represents a groundbreaking effort to use a specific population-based screening programme as an entry into health insurance for low-income populations. It has the potential of providing earlier treatment and, furthermore, expanded health benefits to millions of previously uninsured and underinsured women. Currently, the federal government had approved this expansion for 49 states. In 2002, the Bush administration authorised Medicare coverage for the treatment of Alzheimer's disease, which afflicts nearly 4 million Americans. Medicare beneficiaries will now receive reimbursement for the costs of mental health services, hospice care or home health care (Pear 2002). In addition, several states have begun to make prescription drugs more affordable to low-income and elderly Americans (Department of Health and Human Services 2002).

Conclusions

Access to health care is a growing and significant problem in the United States. Following a dramatic transformation of the health care delivery system in recent years, more Americans are finding it harder to access, and pay for, the health care services they need to improve their health outcomes. Providers of both public and private health care services are faced with increasing costs and other related barriers that result in decreased access to care for consumers.

The greatest influence on access to care is health care insurance. While some efforts have been made to expand health care coverage in the United States, the reality is that significant inequalities still exist. The inequities described in this chapter are fuelled by dramatic differences in health insurance coverage. Ethnic minorities, as well as women, tend to have worse health outcomes because of the lack of access to affordable health care coverage. These groups are more likely to be uninsured, to forgo needed health care, and to rely on an inconsistent system of safety net providers.

Universal access, once considered a novel idea and a political impossibility, has re-emerged as a possible solution to the health care crisis in America. Groups like Physicians for a National Health Program, as well as politicians and advocates, are calling for a national programme to provide comprehensive health care to all Americans. As best-selling author and political columnist Molly Ivins wrote recently, 'if you don't have health insurance, the system is an insane nightmare' (Ivins 2002: page 1). Only time will tell if the United States will wake up from the nightmare and realise that providing equal access to health care is not only possible but critical for the health of all Americans.

References

Aday, L., Begley, C., Lairson, D. and Slater, C. (1993) *Evaluating the Medical Care System: Effectiveness, Efficiency, and Equity*. Ann Arbor: Health Administration Press.

American Cancer Society (2002) *Breast Cancer Facts and Figures: 2001–2002*. Atlanta: American Cancer Society.

American College of Physicians/American Society of Internal Medicine (2000) *No Health Insurance? It's Enough to Make You Sick*. Philadelphia, PA: American College of Physicians/American Society of Internal Medicine. http://www.acponline.org/uninsured/ ; accessed 18 September 2002.

American Hospital Association (2000) 'Essential access: broadening the safety net', *AHA Trend Watch*, 2(2).

American Hospital Association (2001) *Hospital Statistics 2001 Edition*. Chicago, IL: Health Forum, LLC.

Asplin, B.R. (2001) 'Tying a knot in the unraveling health care safety net', *Academic Emergency Medicine*, 8: 1075–9.

Ayanian, J.Z., Kohler, B.A., Abe, T. and Epstein, A.M. (1993) 'The relation between health insurance coverage and clinical outcomes among women with breast cancer', *New England Journal of Medicine*, 329: 326–31.

Ayanian, J.Z., Weissman, J.S., Schneider, E.C., Ginsburg, J.A. and Zaslavsky, A.M. (2000) 'Unmet health needs of uninsured adults in the United States', *Journal of the American Medical Association*, 284: 2061–9.

Bindman, A.B., Grumbach, K., Osmond, D., Vranizan, K. and Stewart, A.L (1996) 'Primary care and receipt of preventive services', *Journal of General Internal Medicine*, 11: 269–76.

Bodenheimer, T (1992) 'Underinsurance in America', *The New England Journal of Medicine*, 327: 4.

Boyer-Chammard, A., Taylor, T.H. and Anton-Culver, H. (1999) 'Survival differences in breast cancer among racial/ethnic groups: A population-based study', *Cancer Detection and Prevention*, 23: 463–73.

Bradley, C.J., Given, C.W. and Roberts, C. (2002) 'Race, socioeconomic status, and breast cancer treatment and survival', *Journal of the National Cancer Institute*, 94: 490–6.

Bureau of Health Professions (1993) *Ninth Report to Congress: Health Personnel in the United States. Health Resource and Services Administration*. Washington, DC: US Department of Health and Human Services, DHHS Publication No. P-OD-94-1.

Centers for Disease Control and Prevention (2001) *Health, United States*. Washington, DC: Department of Health and Human Services. National Center for Health Statistics.

Centers for Medicare and Medicaid Services (2002) *Programs. Medicare*. Baltimore, MD: Centers for Medicare and Medicaid Services. http://cms.hhs.gov/about/programs.asp; accessed 18 September 2002.

Claxton, G. (2002) *How Private Insurance Works: A Primer*. Prepared for the Henry J. Kaiser Family Foundation. Washington, DC: Georgetown University Institution for Health Care Research and Policy.

Collins, K.S., Schoen, C., Joseph, S., Duchon, L., Simantov, E. and Yellowitz, M. (1999) *Health Concerns Across a Woman's Lifespan*. New York: The Commonwealth Fund.

Collins, K.S., Hughes, D.L., Doty, M.M., Ives, B.L., Edwards, H.N. and Tenney, K. (2001) *Diverse Communities, Common Concerns: Assessing Health Care Quality for Minority Americans*. New York: The Commonwealth Fund.

Congressional Budget Office (1997a) *Trends in Health Care Spending by the Private Sector.* Washington, DC: Congressional Budget Office.

Congressional Budget Office (1997b) *Testimony on Baseline Projections for Medicare and Medicaid.* Washington, DC: Congressional Budget Office.

Council on Graduate Medical Education (1998) *Tenth Report: Physician Distribution and Health Care Challenges in Rural and Inner-City Areas.* Washington, DC: US Department of Health and Human Services, Public Health Service.

Cullen, T., Hart, L., Whitcomb, M. and Rosenblatt, R. (1997) 'The National Health Service Corps: rural physician service and retention', *Journal of the American Board of Family Practictioners*, 10: 272–9.

Cunningham, P.J. and Kemper, P. (1998) 'Ability to obtain medical care for the uninsured: how much does it vary across communities?', *Journal of the American Medical Association*, 280: 921–7.

Cunningham, W.E. Andersen, R.M., Katz, M.H., Stein, M.D., Turner, B.J., Crystal, S., Zierler, S., Kuromiya, K., Morton, S.C., St Clair, P., Bozzette, S.A. and Shapiro, M.F. (1999) 'The impact of competing subsistence needs and barriers on access to medical care for persons with human immunodeficiency virus receiving care in the United States', *Medical Care*, 37: 1270–81.

Current Population Survey (CPS) (2001) *Health Insurance Coverage 2000.* Washington, DC: United States Census Bureau.

DeLew, N., Greenberg, G. and Kinchen, K. (1992) 'A layman's guide to the U.S. health care system', *Health Care Financing Review*, 14: 151–69.

Department of Health and Human Services (2002) HHS approves demonstration projects in Minnesota, Georgia to expand safety-net patients' access to prescription drugs. Washington, DC: Department of Health and Human Services. http://www.hhs.gov/news/press/2002pres/20020401a.html; accessed 18 September 2002.

Derickson, A. (2002) 'Health for three-thirds of the nation', *American Journal of Public Health*, 92: 180–90.

Dewar, H. and Goldstein, A. (2002) 'Democrats trim prescription drug plans, senators seek proposal for Medicare recipients that can attract GOP votes', *The Washington Post*, 28 July.

Families USA (2001) *New Report: Over 725,000 Laid-off Workers Lost Health Coverage Since Recession Began in March: 345,000 Lost Health Coverage in September and October.* Washington, DC: Families USA. http://www.familiesusa.org/media/pdf/cobra.pdf; accessed 18 September 2002.

Fehr-Snyder, K. (2002) 'Hospitals lack interpreters', *The Arizona Republic*, 9 January 2002.

Felt-Lisk, S., Dodge, R. and McHugh, M. (2001) *Trend in health plans servicing Medicaid: 2000 Data Update.* Prepared for The Kaiser Commission on Medicaid and the Uninsured, Washington, DC: Mathmatica Policy Research, Inc.

Fiscella, K., Franks, P., Doescher, M.P. and Saver, B.G. (2002) 'Disparities in health care by race, ethnicity, and language among the insured: findings from a national sample', *Medical Care*, 40: 52–9.

Flores, G. (2000) 'Culture and the patient–physician relationship: achieving cultural competency in health care', *Journal of Pediatrics*, 136: 14–23.

Flores, G., Abreu, M., Olivar, M.A. and Kastner, B. (1998) 'Access barriers to health care for Latino children', *Archives of Pediatrics and Adolescent Medicine*, 152: 1119–25.

Government Accounting Office (1997) *Private Health Insurance: Continued Erosion of Coverage Linked to Cost Pressures.* Washington, DC: GAO/HEHS-97–122.

Government Accounting Office (1998) *Private Health Insurance: Employer Coverage Trends Signal Possible Decline in Access for 55–64 Year-Olds.* Washington, DC: GAO/T-HEHS-98–199.

Government Accounting Office (2001a) *Private Health Insurance: Small Employees Continue to Face Challenges in Providing Coverage,* Washington, DC: GAO-02-8.

Government Accounting Office (2001b) *Health Insurance: Characteristics and Trends in the Uninsured Population.* Washington, DC: GAO-01-507T.

Guidry, J.J., Aday, L.A. and Winn, R.J. (1997) 'Transportation as a barrier to cancer treatment', *Cancer Practice*, 5: 361–6.

Guyer, J., Broaddus, M. and Dude, A. (2002) 'Millions of mothers lack health insurance coverage in the United States. Most uninsured mothers lack access both to employer-based coverage and to publicly subsidized health insurance', *International Journal of Health Services*, 32: 89–106.

Hadley, J. (2002) *Sicker and Poorer: The Consequences of Being Uninsured.* Prepared for The Kaiser Commission on Medicaid and the Uninsured. Washington, DC: The Urban Institute.

Hafner-Eaton, C. (1993) 'Physician utilization disparities between the uninsured and insured: comparisons of the chronically ill, acutely ill, and well non-elderly populations', *Journal of the American Medical Association*, 269: 787–92.

Hart, L.G. (1997) 'Physician staffing ratios in staff-model HMOs: a cautionary tale', *Health Affairs*, 16: 55–70.

Health Services Resources and Services Administration (2000) *United States Health Workforce Personnel Factbook.* Washington, DC: US Department of Health and Human Services.

Herbert, B. (2001) 'The quiet scourge: AIDS is ravaging blacks in America', *The New York Times OP-ED*, Thursday, 11 January: A31.

Hicks, L.L. and Glen, J.K. (1991) 'Rural population and rural physicians: estimates of critical mass ratios, by specialty', *Journal of Rural Health*, 7: 357–72.

Hoffman, C. and Pohl, M.B. (2002) *Health Insurance Coverage in America: 2000 Data Update.* Washington, DC: The Kaiser Commission on Medicaid and the Uninsured.

Holahan, J. (2002) *Health Care Access for Uninsured Adults.* Washington, DC: Urban Institute.

Hudman, J. (2000) *Immigrants' Health: Coverage and Access.* Washington, DC: Kaiser Commission on Medicaid and the Uninsured.

Iglehart, J.K. (1992) 'The American health care system: introduction', *New England Journal of Medicine*, 326: 962–7.

Iglehart, J.K. (1993) 'Health care reform and graduate medical education', *New England Journal of Medicine*, 330: 1167–71.

Iglehart, J.K. (1995) 'Medicaid and managed care', *The New England Journal of Medicine*, 332: 1727–31.

Iglehart, J.K. (1999) 'The American health care system: expenditures', *The New England Journal of Medicine*, 340: 70–6.

Institute of Medicine (2000) *America's Health Care Safety Net: Intact but Endangered.* Washington, DC: National Academy Press.

Institute of Medicine (2002a) *Unequal Treatment: Confronting Racial and Ethnic Disparities in Health Care.* Washington, DC: National Academy Press.

Institute of Medicine (2002b) *Care without Coverage: Too Little Too Late. Committee on the Consequences of Uninsurance, Board on Health Care Services.* Washington, DC: National Academy Press.

Ivins, M. (2002) 'The nation must fix its seriously ailing health care system', *Contra Costa Times*, 28 March.

Kaiser Commission on Medicaid and the Uninsured (2001a) *COBRA Coverage for Low-Income Unemployed Workers.* Washington, DC: Kaiser Commission on Medicaid and the Uninsured.

Kaiser Commission on Medicaid and the Uninsured (2001b) *Health Coverage for Low-Income Children.* Washington, DC: Kaiser Family Foundation.

Kaiser Commission on Medicaid and the Uninsured (2001c) *Medicaid and Managed Care: Key Facts.* Washington, DC: Kaiser Commission on Medicaid and the Uninsured.

Kaiser Commission on Medicaid and the Uninsured (2001d) *Medicare at a Glance.* Washington, DC: Kaiser Commission on Medicaid and the Uninsured.

Kaiser Commission on Medicaid and the Uninsured (2001e) *Immigrants' Health Care Coverage and Access: Key Facts.* Washington, DC: Kaiser Commission on Medicaid and the Uninsured.

Kaiser Commission on Medicaid and the Uninsured (2003) *The Uninsured and Their Access to Health Care: Key Facts.* Washington, DC: Kaiser Commission on Medicaid and the Uninsured.

Kaiser Family Foundation (2002) *Women's Health in the United States: Health Coverage and Access to Care.* Washington, DC: Kaiser Family Foundation.

Ku, L. and Matani, S. (2001) 'Left out: immigrants' access to health care and insurance', *Health Affairs*, 20: 247–56.

Kuttner, R. (1999) 'The American health care system: employer-sponsored health coverage', *The New England Journal of Medicine*, 340: 248–52.

Lambrew, J. (2001) *Diagnosing Disparities In Health Insurance For Women: A Prescription for Change.* Prepared for The Commonwealth Fund. Washington, DC: The George Washington University.

Lee, R.C. (1991) 'Current approaches to shortage area designation', *Journal of Rural Health*, 7: 437–50.

Levitt, L. and Lundy, J. (1998) *Trend and Indicators in the Changing HealthCare Marketplace: Chartbook.* Washington, DC: The Henry J. Kaiser Family Foundation.

Lipson, D. and Naierman, N. (1996) 'Safety-net providers', *Health Affairs*, 15: 33–48

Maloy, K.A., Darnell, J., Nolan, L., Kenney, K.A. and Cyprien, S. (2000) *Effects of the 1996 Welfare and Immigration Reform Laws on the Ability and Willingness of Immigrants to Access Medicaid and Health Care Services.* Washington, DC: George Washington University.

Mann, C., Hudman, J., Salganicoff, A. and Folsom, A. (2002) 'Five years later: poor women's health care coverage after welfare reform', *Journal of the American Medical Women's Association*, 57: 16–22.

Marks, A. (2002) 'Healthcare "crisis" grows for middle class', *Christian Science Monitor*, 3 April.

McAlearney, J.S. (2002) 'The financial performance of community health centers, 1996–1999. Clear evidence that many CHCs are on the brink of financial insolvency', *Health Affairs*, 21: 219–25.

McKinney, M.M. (1998) 'Service needs and networks of rural women with HIV/AIDS', *AIDS Patient Care and Stds*, 12: 471–80.

Miller, J.E. (2001) *A Perfect Storm: The Confluence of Forces Affecting Health Care Coverage*. Washington DC: National Coalition on Health Care.

Mirvis, D.M., Bailey, J.E. and Chang, C.F. (2002) 'TennCare – Medicaid managed care in Tennessee in jeopardy', *American Journal of Managed Care*, 8: 57–68.

Mofidi, M., Rozier, G.R. and King, R.S. (2002) 'Problems with access to dental care for Medicaid-insured children: what caregivers think', *American Journal of Public Health*, 92: 53–8.

Morehouse Medical Treatment and Effectiveness Center (1999) A synthesis of the literature: racial and ethnic disparities in access to Medicare care. Atlanta: The Henry J. Kaiser Family Foundation.

Mouradian, W.E., Wehr, E. and Crall, J.J. (2000) 'Disparities in children's oral health and access to dental care', *Journal of the American Medical Association*, 284: 2625–31.

Mueller, C.D., Schur C.L. and Paramore, L.C. (1998) 'Access to dental care in the United States', *Journal of the American Dental Association*, 129: 429–37.

National Association of Community Health Centers (2002) *A Legacy of Caring: A Commitment to the Future*. Bethesda, MD: National Association of Community Health Centers.

National Center for Health Statistics (1990) *Health United States, 1991, with Chartbook on Trends in the Health of Americans*. DHHS Pub. no. PHS 1-1232. Washington, DC: Government Printing Office.

National Center for Health Statistics (2001) *Health United States, 2001, with Chartbook on Trends in the Health of Americans*. DHHS Pub. no. PHS 1-1232, 1-0237. Washington, DC: Government Printing Office.

National Center for Health Statistics (2002) *Health United States, 2002, with Chartbook on Trends in the Health of Americans*. DHHS Pub. no. PHS 2-1232, 2-0016. Available: http://www.cdc.gov/nchs/about/major/nhis/hisdesc.htm; accessed 18 September 2002.

National Governors Association (2000) *Primer on the Health Care Safety Net*. Washington, DC: National Governors Association.

National Governors Association (2002) *Governors Seek Increase in Federal Share for Medicaid*. Washington, DC: National Governors Association.

National Rural Health Association (1999) *Access to Health Care for the Uninsured in Rural and Frontier America*. Washington, DC: National Rural Health Association.

National Women's Law Center (2001) *Making the Grade on Women's Health: A National and State-by-State Report Card 2001*. Washington, DC: National Women's Law Center.

Office of Minority Health. Department of Health and Human Services (2001) *Assuring Cultural Competence in Health Care: Developing National Standards and an Outcomes-Focused Research Agenda*. Washington, DC: Department of Health and Human Services.

Orloff, T.M. and Tymann, B. (1995) *Rural Health: An Evolving System of Accessible Services*. Washington, DC: Center for Policy Research, National Governors Association.

Pappas, G., Hadden, W.C., Kozak, L.J. and Fisher, G.F. (1997) 'Potentially avoidable hospitalizations: inequalities in rates between US socioeconomic groups', *American Journal of Public Health*, 87: 811–16.

Pear, R. (2002) 'In a first, Medicare coverage is authorized for Alzheimers', *The New York Times*, 31 March.

Politzer, R.M., Harris, M.H. and Mullan, F. (1991) 'Primary care physician supply and the medically underserved: A status report and recommendations', *Journal of the American Medical Association*, 266: 104–8.

Ries, L.A.G., Eisner, M.P., Kosary, C.L., Hankey B.F., Miller, B.A., Clegg, L. and Edwards, B.D. (eds) (2002) *SEER Cancer Statistics Review, 1973–1999*. Bethesda, MD: National Cancer Institute.

Rosenbaum, S., Stewart, A. and Sonosky, C. (2002) *Negotiating the New Health System. A Nationwide Study of Medicaid Managed Care Contacts, Fourth Edition*. Washington, DC: Center for Health Services Research and Policy, George Washington University. Available online only at: www.gwhealthpolicy.org.

Rosenblatt, R.A. and Lishner, D.M. (1991) 'Surplus or shortage? Unraveling the physician supply conundrum', *Western Journal of Medicine*, 154: 43–50.

Rowland, D. (2002) 'The new challenge of the uninsured: coverage in the new economy'. Testimony presented on 28 February 2002 for the Subcommittee on Health, Committee on Energy and Commerce, US House of Representatives. Printed by the Kaiser Commission on Medicaid and the Uninsured.

Schneider, E.C., Zaslavsky, A.M. and Epstein, A.M. (2002) 'Racial disparities in the quality of care for enrollees in Medicare managed care', *Journal of the American Medical Association*, 287(10): 1288–94.

Schoen, C. (2001) *Security Matters: How Instability in Health Insurance Puts U.S. Workers at Risk*. New York: The Commonwealth Fund.

Smith, V.K. (2002) *Making Medicaid Better: Options to Allow State to Continue to Participate and to Bring the Program Up to Date in Today's Health Care Marketplace*. Washington, DC: Health Management Association. Prepared for the National Governors Association.

Star, P. (1992) *The Social Transformation of American Medicine*. New York: Basic Books.

Strunk, B.C. and Cunningham, P.J. (2002) *Treading Water: Americans' Access to Needed Medical Care, 1997–2001*. Princeton, NJ: Center for Studying Health System Change.

Sultz, H.A. and Young, K.M. (1997) *Health Care USA: Understanding its Organization and Delivery*. Gaithersburg: Aspen Publications.

United States Department of Health and Human Services. Bureau of Health Professions http://www.bhpr.hrsa.gov/. accessed 22 October 2002.

Waitzman, H., Williams, R.L., McCloskey, J. and Wagner, W. (2002) 'Safety-net institutions buffer the impact of Medicaid managed care: a multi-method assessment in a rural state', *American Journal of Public Health*, 92: 598–610.

Weitzman, M. (1997) 'Health care for children of immigrant families', *Pediatrics*, 100: 153–4.

Wilensky, G.R. (1995) 'Incremental health system reform: where Medicare fits in', *Health Affairs*, 14: 173–81.

Wilensky, G.R. (2001) 'Medicare reform: now is the time', *New England Journal of Medicine*, 345: 458–62.

Chapter 8

Access to health care in the European Union
The impact of user charges and voluntary health insurance

Elias Mossialos and Sarah Thomson

Introduction

Universal or near universal rights to health care can be found in every member state of the European Union (EU).[1] It is widely acknowledged, however, that universal rights do not automatically ensure universal access to health care (Glennerster *et al.* 2000). In recognition of existing barriers to access in the health care systems of many member states, and in support of community-wide action to remove such barriers, the European Commission recently proposed the achievement of universal access to health care as a common objective of EU health care systems and a priority objective for EU co-operation in social protection (European Commission 1999; European Commission 2001). The Commission's proposal follows recent attempts by some member states to increase access to health care, one notable attempt being the introduction of universal health insurance coverage in France in 2000. The proposal also reflects policy debates about widening access to health care in other countries, such as the Swedish government's joint initiative with governments in the United Kingdom (UK), Chile, Germany, Greece, New Zealand and Slovenia to promote solidarity in health care systems (Ministry of Health and Social Affairs 2002).

For the purpose of this chapter we adopt a more restricted definition of access to health care in terms of 'the actual use of personal health services and everything that facilitates or impedes that use' (Andersen 1995). From an economic perspective, barriers to access are associated with supply-side factors, such as the existence of a statutory system of health insurance, the level of public financial resources for health care, the level of human resources for health care, the allocation of these resources, the location of health services and the existence of waiting times for treatment. Supply-side factors broadly relate to service availability, relevance and effectiveness. They may be financial or organisational in nature and will present barriers to access either as a result of scarcity (insufficient resources) or as a result of unacceptable variations in supply (unequal distribution of resources). While financial factors affect the supply of health services, organisational barriers are often caused by capacity issues and have implications for the timeliness and acceptability of health services (Gulliford *et al.* 2001).

Demand-side factors can also restrict access to health care (Kasper 2000). For example, individuals' ability to pay for health services (income) and other personal characteristics (knowledge, beliefs, information, preferences and opportunity costs) are likely to influence their use of health services. Demand-side barriers may therefore be financial, socio-economic, psycho-social or socio-cultural in nature. The existence of a barrier to access often depends on the complex interaction of supply- and demand-side factors, and both types of factor will determine the extent to which access to health care is equitable; that is, based on the principle of equal utilisation for equal need.

In this chapter we focus on financial barriers to access in the European Union. We begin by briefly outlining recent initiatives to reduce both organisational and financial barriers to access, including a discussion of statutory health insurance coverage. We go on to explore the implications of a gradual process of 'de-insurance' for access to health care in different member states. Specifically, we examine the financial barriers to access posed by increasing reliance on private funds for health care. We assess the extent to which the imposition of statutory user charges and the existence of different types of voluntary health insurance (VHI)[2] deter individuals from using health services and whether they result in health care systems characterised by unequal utilisation for equal need. As much as our choice of focus here is determined by the constraints of a single chapter, it is equally determined by the relative and increasing importance of these financial barriers to access across the European Union.

Initiatives to reduce barriers to access in the European Union

Some barriers to access are common to every member state in the European Union; others are more country-specific. Recent policy responses to problems of access to health care have ranged from addressing organisational barriers, such as the introduction of waiting time guarantees and the enactment of patients' rights legislation, to attempts to remove financial barriers through the improvement of resource allocation mechanisms and the expansion of statutory health insurance coverage.

During the 1990s several member states introduced initiatives aimed at reducing waiting lists, with mixed results. Waiting time guarantees introduced in Denmark, Sweden and the United Kingdom were initially successful in reducing waiting lists, but were unable to sustain these reductions in the longer term (Hanning 1996; Hanning and Spångberg 2000). There is also evidence to suggest that the initiatives led to increased waiting times in other areas, at least in Denmark and the United Kingdom (Newton et al. 1995; Christensen et al. 1999; Harrison 2000).

Finland and Greece enshrined patients' rights in law at the beginning of the 1990s (World Health Organization 2000a). Following on from the World Health Organization's 1994 'Amsterdam Declaration' promoting patients' rights, Denmark, Finland and the Netherlands have also enacted patients' rights legislation

(Fallberg 2000a). France, Ireland, Portugal and the United Kingdom use non-legal frameworks (patients' charters) to promote the rights of patients (Fallberg 2000a). Measures to promote and enforce patients' rights are to be welcomed, particularly in so far as they provide a framework for protecting the needs of marginalised social groups, but it is important to acknowledge that legislation and non-legal frameworks do not in themselves guarantee change. As one commentator has observed, 'in [some EU member states], where laws on the rights of patients have been introduced during the last decade, experience shows that legislation doesn't necessarily change the behaviour of health services personnel' (Fallberg 2000a: 1). Moreover, patients' rights legislation in the European Union is rarely comprehensive, often covering some, but not all, rights. For example, the 1998 Danish Patients' Rights Act aims to safeguard patients' autonomy, rather than securing material rights to treatment (World Health Organization 2000b). Conversely, the equivalent Finnish legislation lacks regulations concerning patients' autonomy, but does guarantee the right to treatment (Fallberg 2000b; World Health Organization 2000b). However, the guarantee is not absolute and can be limited by the availability of resources. Gaps in public knowledge about the existence of patients' rights also need to be filled (World Health Organization 2000b).

Elsewhere, efforts have been made to increase equity in the distribution of financial resources for health care, for example by introducing or refining mechanisms to allocate resources to geographically-defined populations (in tax-funded health care systems) or sickness funds (in social health insurance systems). The resource allocation formula used in England was adapted in 1995 to take into account inequalities in health, while in 1992 a new formula was introduced in the Stockholm area in Sweden, with the aim of allocating proportionately more resources to populations with poorer health and socio-economic characteristics (Diderichsen *et al.* 1997; Rice and Smith 2002). Since the introduction of competition between sickness funds in the Netherlands in 1988 and in Germany in 1996, sickness funds in both countries have been subject to risk adjustment mechanisms. The risk adjustment scheme in the Netherlands adjusts for age, sex, region, employment and disability status; the German scheme is based on income and average expenditure by age and sex (Busse 2001; Okma and Poelert 2001).

The introduction of universal coverage in France is perhaps the most significant recent attempt to increase access to health care in the European Union. In 1999 the French government passed a law on universal health coverage (*Couverture Maladie Universelle* – CMU) to enable those who did not benefit from any health insurance to be covered by a compulsory, statutory health insurance scheme (see the section on voluntary health insurance and access to health care below) (Girard and Merlière 2001).

France now joins Denmark, Finland, Greece, Ireland, Italy, Luxembourg, Portugal, Sweden and the United Kingdom in providing universal statutory health coverage (Organisation for Economic Co-operation and Development 2001). Near universal coverage can be found in Austria (99 per cent), Belgium (99 per cent)[3]

Table 8.1 Percentage of the population covered by the statutory health care system in EU member states, 1960–97

Country	Type of care	1960	1970	1980	1990	1997
Austria	Total	78.0	91.0	99.0	99.0	99.0
Belgium	Inpatient	58.0	97.8	99.0	97.3	99.0
	Outpatient	58.0	93.0	93.0	93.0	94.0
Denmark	Total	95.0	100.0	100.0	100.0	100.0
Finland	Inpatient	55.0	100.0	100.0	100.0	100.0
	Outpatient	100.0	100.0	100.0	100.0	100.0
France	Total	76.3	95.7	99.3	99.5	99.5
Germany	Total	85.0	88.0	91.0	92.2	92.2
Greece	Inpatient	30.0	55.0	88.0	100.0	100.0
	Outpatient	75.0	90.0	97.0	100.0	n/a
Ireland	Inpatient	85.0	85.0	100.0	100.0	100.0
	Outpatient	30.0	30.0	35.0	37.0	32.9
Italy	Total	87.0	93.0	100.0	100.0	100.0
Luxembourg	Inpatient	90.0	100.0	100.0	100.0	100.0
	Outpatient	100.0	100.0	100.0	100.0	n/a
Netherlands	Inpatient	71.0	n/a	74.6	73.9	74.6
	Outpatient	71.0	72.0	72.2	72.5	72.7
Portugal	Total	18.0	40.0	100.0	100.0	100.0
Spain	Total	54.0	61.0	83.0	99.0	99.8
Sweden	Total	100.0	100.0	100.0	100.0	100.0
UK	Total	100.0	100.0	100.0	100.0	100.0

Source: OECD (Organisation for Economic Co-operation and Development 2001).

and Spain (99.8 per cent). Table 8.1 shows the increase in levels of coverage in all member states since 1960.

Statutory health coverage is lowest in Germany (92.2 per cent in 1997) and the Netherlands (74.2 per cent in 1999). About 5 per cent of the German population chooses to obtain protection through the purchase of substitutive VHI rather than contribute to the statutory health insurance scheme, but everyone is covered by mandatory insurance for long-term care (Busse 2000).[4] Even in the Netherlands, where a significant percentage of the population is excluded from participating in the statutory health insurance scheme for primary care and acute inpatient care (currently those earning over €30,700 a year), all legal residents are compulsorily covered for long-term care, including stays in hospital that are longer than one year, mental health care and care for disabled people (Ministry of Health Welfare and Sport 2002). In both countries the percentage of the population without any type of health insurance is low (less than 0.2 per cent in Germany and 1.25 per cent in the Netherlands); the uninsured in the Netherlands are mainly homeless people or those who conscientiously object to insurance (Busse 2000; Ministry of Health Welfare and Sport 2000).

In spite of the official achievement of universal or near universal statutory health coverage, there are persistent problems of access associated with the gaps in coverage that do remain. These problems arise in two ways: as a consequence of the exclusion of particular treatments or whole areas of treatment from statutory health coverage, or as a consequence of increasing reliance on patient cost sharing through user charges.

Over the last two decades, the most common areas of treatment to be fully or partially excluded from statutory health coverage are dental care and pharmaceuticals, which have been removed from positive lists of benefits, placed on negative lists or become chargeable services. In almost all member states patients must now make out-of-pocket payments for dental care and/or pharmaceuticals, or purchase complementary VHI to cover the cost of these and other health services.

Although health care systems in the European Union are still characterised by a high degree of public expenditure, the last twenty years have seen some decline in levels of public expenditure as a proportion of total expenditure on health care (see Table 8.2).

Out-of-pocket payments have traditionally accounted for a substantial proportion of health care expenditure in member states such as Greece, Italy, Portugal and Spain (see Table 8.3). While data on private spending should be treated with some caution, particularly with regard to health care systems in which informal payments are a common feature, it is accurate to note that private expenditure grew substantially as a proportion of total expenditure on health care in Austria, Denmark and the United Kingdom in the 1980s, and in Finland, Italy, Luxembourg and Spain during the 1990s. As a result, out-of-pocket payments are now the dominant source of private expenditure on health care in every member state except France and the Netherlands (see Table 8.3).[5]

Spending on VHI as a proportion of private expenditure is relatively low, however, accounting for less than 5 per cent in Greece, Italy and Portugal and for less than 25 per cent in Austria, Belgium, Denmark, Finland, Luxembourg, Spain and the United Kingdom. This can be attributed to the fact that governments have tended to rely on other methods of shifting health care costs onto consumers. The preference has generally been for imposing user charges over and above promoting and subsidising VHI.

Significant increases in the proportion of private expenditure on health care during the 1980s and 1990s, most notably in Denmark, Finland, Germany, Ireland, Italy, Sweden and the United Kingdom, suggest that the achievement of universal rights to health care, in terms of universal coverage, has been accompanied by a process of selective 'de-insurance'. That is to say, at the same time as statutory health insurance has been extended to cover the whole population, the comprehensiveness of this cover has declined, lowering its protective value to the individual.

It has been clearly established that private expenditure produces inequity in health care funding because it shifts the funding burden away from population-based risk-pooling arrangements, in which people contribute through taxation or social health insurance on the basis of their ability to pay, towards out-of-pocket payments by individuals and households, with a pro-rich distributive impact (Evans and Barer 1995; Creese 1997). The higher the proportion of private expenditure in the total mix of funding for health care, the greater the relative share of the

Table 8.2 Public and private expenditure as a percentage of total expenditure on health care in the European Union, 1975–98

Country		1975	1980	1985	1990	1995	1996	1997	1998	Overall growth 1975–90 (%)	Overall growth 1990–98 (%)
Austria	public	69.6	73.7	68.1	66.1	71.8	70.5	70.9	70.6	-5.3	6.8
	private	30.4	26.3	31.9	33.9	28.2	29.5	29.1	29.4	10.3	-13.3
Belgium	public	79.6	83.4	81.8	88.9	88.7	88.8	89.3	89.7	10.5	0.9
	private	20.4	16.6	18.2	11.1	11.3	11.2	10.7	10.3	-83.8	-7.2
Denmark	public	–	87.8	85.6	82.6	82.5	82.4	82.4	81.9	-5.9	-0.8
	private	–	12.2	14.4	17.4	17.5	17.6	17.6	18.1	42.6	4.0
Finland	public	78.6	79.0	78.7	80.9	75.6	75.8	76.0	75.9	2.8	-6.2
	private	21.4	21.0	21.3	19.1	24.4	24.2	24.0	24.1	-12.0	26.2
France	public	77.2	78.8	83.4	76.9	76.3	76.3	76.3	76.4	-0.4	-0.7
	private	22.8	21.2	16.6	23.1	23.7	23.7	23.7	23.6	1.3	2.2
Germany	public	79.0	78.6	77.4	76.3	78.0	78.3	76.9	–	-3.5	0.8
	private	21.0	21.4	22.6	23.7	22.0	21.7	23.1	–	11.4	-2.5
Greece	public	–	55.6	–	62.7	58.7	58.7	57.7	56.8	12.8	-9.4
	private	–	44.4	–	37.3	41.3	41.3	42.3	43.2	-16.0	15.8
Ireland	public	79.0	81.6	75.7	71.7	72.7	72.5	75.0	75.8	-10.2	5.7
	private	21.0	18.4	24.3	28.3	27.3	27.5	25.0	24.2	25.8	-14.5
Italy	public	84.5	80.5	77.2	78.1	67.7	67.8	68.0	68.0	-8.2	-12.9
	private	15.5	19.5	22.8	21.9	32.3	32.2	32.0	32.0	29.2	46.1
Luxembourg	public	91.8	91.2	89.4	93.1	92.5	–	91.0	92.3	1.4	-0.9
	private	8.2	8.8	10.6	6.9	7.5	–	9.0	7.7	-18.8	11.6
Netherlands	public	69.5	71.1	72.8	68.7	72.5	67.7	69.7	74.7	-1.2	8.7
	private	30.5	28.9	27.2	31.3	27.5	32.3	30.3	25.3	2.6	-19.2
Portugal	public	58.9	64.3	54.4	52.9	54.0	64.2	66.7	66.9	-11.3	26.5
	private	41.1	35.7	45.6	47.1	46.0	35.8	33.3	33.1	12.7	-29.7
Spain	public	77.4	79.9	81.1	78.7	78.3	78.5	76.5	76.9	1.7	-2.3
	private	22.6	20.1	18.9	21.3	21.7	21.5	23.5	23.1	-6.1	8.5
Sweden	public	90.2	92.5	90.4	89.9	85.2	84.8	84.3	83.8	-0.3	-6.8
	private	9.8	7.5	9.6	10.1	14.8	15.2	15.7	16.2	3.0	60.4
UK	public	–	90.1	86.0	86.0	85.8	83.8	83.6	85.7	-4.6	-0.3
	private	–	9.9	14.0	14.0	14.2	16.2	16.4	14.3	41.4	2.1

Source: OECD (Organisation for Economic Co-operation and Development 2001)

Table 8.3 Breakdown of private expenditure as a percentage of total expenditure on health care in the European Union, 1980–98

Country		1980	1985	1990	1995	1996	1997	1998	Overall growth 1980–90 (%)[1]	Overall growth 1990–98 (%)[1]
Austria	VHI	7.6	9.8	9.0	7.8	7.2	7.5	7.1	18.4	–21.1
	OOP[2]	16.3	19.6	22.4	14.8	15.9	17.7	18.3	37.4	–18.3
	Other[3]	2.4	2.5	2.5	5.6	6.4	3.9	4.0	4.2	60.0
Belgium	VHI	0.8	1.2	1.6	1.9	2.0	–	–	100.0	25.0
	OOP	15.8	17.0	9.5	9.4	9.2	–	–	–39.9	–3.2
Denmark	VHI non-profit	0.8	0.8	1.3	1.2	1.4	1.4	1.5	62.5	15.4
	OOP	11.4	13.6	16.1	16.3	16.2	16.2	16.6	41.2	3.1
Finland	VHI non-profit	0.6	0.6	0.5	0.4	–	–	0.5	–16.7	0.0
	VHI for-profit	0.8	1.2	1.7	2.0	–	–	2.2	112.5	29.4
	VHI total	1.4	1.8	2.2	2.4	2.4	2.5	2.7	57.1	22.7
	OOP	18.4	18.3	15.5	20.5	20.2	19.9	19.8	–15.8	27.7
	Other	1.2	1.2	1.4	1.5	1.6	1.6	1.6	16.7	14.3
France	VHI non-profit	–	5.8	6.8	7.5	–	–	7.8	17.2	14.7
	VHI for-profit	–	–	4.4	4.2	–	–	4.4	–	0.0
	VHI total	–	5.8	11.2	11.7	12.1	12.1	12.2	93.1	8.9
	OOP	–	10.8	10.8	10.9	10.6	10.5	10.3	0.0	–4.6
	Other	–	–	1.1	1.1	1.0	1.1	1.1	–	0.0
Germany	VHI	5.9	6.5	7.2	6.7	6.5	6.9	–	22.0	–4.2
	OOP	10.3	11.2	11.1	10.9	11.0	11.9	–	7.8	7.2
	Other	5.2	4.9	5.4	4.4	4.2	4.3	–	3.8	–20.4
Greece	VHI	–	–	0.9	–	–	–	–	–	–
	OOP	–	–	36.4	–	–	–	–	–	–
Ireland	VHI non-profit	–	9.9	13.9	15.0	–	–	9.4	40.4	–32.4
	OOP	–	14.4	14.4	12.3	–	–	14.8	0.0	2.8
Italy	VHI	0.2	0.5	0.9	1.3	–	1.3	–	350.0	44.4
	OOP	19.3	22.3	21.0	31.0	–	30.7	–	8.8	46.2

continued…

Table 8.3 continued

Country		1980	1985	1990	1995	1996	1997	1998	Overall growth 1980–90 (%)[1]	Overall growth 1990–98 (%)[1]
Luxembourg	VHI non-profit	1.6	1.4	1.4	1.3	–	1.6	–	–12.5	14.3
	OOP	7.2	9.2	5.5	6.2	7.2	7.4	–	–23.6	34.5
Netherlands	VHI non-profit	–	–	–	–	–	–	6.0	–	–3.3
	VHI for-profit	–	11.2	12.1	–	–	–	11.7	8.0	46.3
	VHI total	–	11.2	12.1	–	23.3	22.1	17.7	8.0	–23.4
	OOP	–	–	–	–	7.7	6.6	5.9	–	30.8
	Other	–	–	–	–	1.3	1.6	1.7	–	
Portugal	VHI	–	0.2	0.8	1.4	1.7	–	–	300.0	112.5
	OOP	–	45.4	46.3	44.6	34.1	33.3	–	2.0	–28.1
Spain	VHI	3.2	3.7	3.7	5.2	–	1.5	–	15.6	–59.5
	OOP	–	–	–	16.5	21.5	22.0	–		33.3
UK	VHI	1.3	2.5	3.3	3.2	5.1	5.4	3.5	153.8	6.1
	OOP	8.6	11.5	10.7	11.0	11.1	11.0	10.8	24.4	0.9

Source: OECD (Organisation for Economic Co-operation and Development 2001).

Notes:

No data were available for Sweden.

1 Or nearest year for which data are available.

2 OOP refers to out-of-pocket expenditure.

3 Other refers to health expenditure incurred by corporations and private employers providing occupational health services and other non-funded medical benefits to employees plus expenditure by non-profit institutions serving households (excluding social insurance) such as the Red Cross, philanthropic and charitable institutions, religious orders and lay institutions.

funding burden falling on poor people and people in poor health, reducing solidarity between rich and poor and healthy and unhealthy (van de Ven 1983; Rice and Morrison 1994). International comparisons of progressivity in health care funding consistently find that health care systems that rely heavily on private funding are more regressive than those in which funding is predominantly public (Wagstaff *et al.* 1992; Wagstaff *et al.* 1999).[6] However, even in health care systems that are progressive or proportionate overall, the imposition of user charges or the need for VHI may create financial barriers to access (see below). In the following sections we aim to assess the extent to which private expenditure in the form of user charges and VHI produces inequity in access to health care.

User charges and access to health care

User charges in the European Union

User charges (or co-payments) are employed in all member states to control expenditure on pharmaceuticals. Although most health care in the European Union is publicly funded (see Table 8.2), this is not the case in the pharmaceutical sector, where levels of private expenditure are often high. Pharmaceutical expenditure is predominantly private in Belgium, Finland, Greece and Italy (Organisation for Economic Co-operation and Development 2001). In Denmark it is equally shared between private and public sources of funding. Recently, the share of public expenditure on pharmaceuticals has fallen in several member states, largely in an attempt to contain health care costs (Mossialos and Le Grand 1999). Between 1980 and 1997 the public share of total expenditure on pharmaceuticals declined in nine out of fifteen member states. The decline was small in Sweden, the Netherlands, Portugal and the United Kingdom, but substantial in Italy and Belgium. Conversely, some countries saw an increase in the share of public expenditure on pharmaceuticals – a significant increase in Ireland, a more modest one elsewhere.

In addition to co-payments for pharmaceuticals, every member state makes use of co-payments to control expenditure on dental care (Robinson 2002). Some member states have also introduced co-payments to contain the costs of ambulatory and inpatient services (for example, Austria, Belgium, Finland, France, Ireland, Luxembourg and Sweden), by either raising existing charges or introducing charges for services previously provided free of charge.

Member states generally use three types of co-payment: flat-rate payments that are fixed fees per service, co-insurance based on a percentage of the total cost, and deductibles, which require the user to bear a fixed quantity of the cost, with any excess borne by statutory health insurance. Deductibles can apply to specific cases or for a period of time (usually a year, as in Finland and Sweden).

The proportion of the cost that patients must pay for pharmaceuticals varies by type of drug in France, Greece, Italy and Portugal, and by class of drug in Belgium. Drug co-payments in Germany vary according to pack size, while a flat rate is charged for all drugs in the United Kingdom and Austria, and for some drugs in Belgium. In Belgium, Greece, France, Luxembourg, Portugal and Spain the patient pays a fixed proportion of the cost. Deductibles are used in Denmark, Finland and Sweden (Hjortsberg and Ghatnekar 2001; Järvelin 2002).

Significant population groups are exempt from co-payments in many member states, which limits the impact of user charges as a means of containing health care costs or as a revenue-generating measure (see below). Reduced charges or exemptions for those on low incomes and for other categories of people (for example, pensioners, pregnant women or chronically ill people) vary between member states. Austria, Belgium, Denmark, Finland, Germany, Ireland and Sweden have introduced income protection schemes by setting an annual ceiling on co-payments for some services (Robinson 2002). Many member states exempt children from co-payments for preventive dental care. Exemptions from prescription drug co-payments commonly relate to clinical condition and level of income; some systems also employ age-related criteria (Mossialos and Le Grand 1999; Noyce et al. 2000). Denmark, Ireland and Spain exempt chronically ill people from pharmaceutical co-payments. In Belgium, France, Italy and Portugal drugs are assigned different charges according to whether they are classified as 'essential' or not.[7]

Exemptions may reduce the regressivity of co-payments if they are means tested. However, if exemptions are based on factors other than income, such as age or disease, they may result in horizontal inequity.[8] In Sweden, for example, the pharmaceutical deductible applies to everyone except people suffering from diabetes mellitus, a practice that raises serious equity issues, particularly for young, unemployed or elderly people and single parent households (Hjortsberg and Ghatnekar 2001).

Arguments for and against user charges

Why do so many governments impose user charges for statutory health services? Advocates of user charges claim that they achieve two objectives. It is argued that user charges reduce demand by encouraging a more 'responsible' use of health services. If the cost of a service to users is zero, then users will have an incentive to consume more services than is socially beneficial. User charges therefore prevent health services from being undervalued and abused. This argument is particularly pertinent where governments are concerned about containing health care expenditure. It is also argued that user charges can raise revenue to sustain and expand the provision of health care (Abel-Smith 1994; Chalkley and Robinson 1997; Kutzin 1998; Willman 1998). Any additional revenue raised could be targeted at poor people, spent on tackling inequality in the health care system or used to bridge the funding gap when public budgets are under pressure.

Whether these objectives are achieved in practice depends on different assumptions about the elasticity of demand.[9] If the first objective (reducing demand) is achieved, then the second (raising revenue) cannot be (Towse 1999). Furthermore, if user charges are introduced to raise revenue, then the cost of collecting them must be less than the revenue raised. In practice, the revenue-raising potential of user charges is often severely affected by the exemption of particular groups and by the high cost of administering such exemptions (van de Ven 1983; Rice and Morrison 1994; Evans and Barer 1995). It may also be affected by reluctance on the part of providers to enforce charges due to the additional bureaucracy and corresponding administrative costs involved, as has been the case in Portugal and Greece (Pereira *et al.* 1999; Sissouras *et al.* 1999).

Meanwhile, the experience of the United Kingdom suggests that any savings from primary care charges (such as prescription charges or charges for eye tests and dental check-ups) have often been directed away from improvements in primary care, either to the acute sector or to areas outside the health care system (Eversley and Webster 1997). The additional income may even pave the way for tax cuts, which typically benefit richer people (Eversley and Webster 1997).

Finally, user charges may prove to be an ineffective method of containing health care costs, because they operate on the demand side, whereas health care expenditure is primarily driven by supply-side factors (Evans and Barer 1995). A number of studies have noted that the introduction of user charges for certain health services in Finland, Germany, Spain and Sweden did not lead to stable or lower levels of spending on those services (Lamata 1995; Persson and Guzelgun 1998; Busse 1999; Häkkinen 1999). The imperfect information possessed by patients means that many decisions regarding the use of services are made by doctors and are not based on patients' individual assessment of likely benefits. Therefore, if the objective is to reduce demand, it would be more appropriate to charge patients for services that they initiate themselves. Also, the assertion that charges will deter the unnecessary use of health services assumes that people can always tell whether a product or service is unnecessary.

Do user charges have a detrimental effect on the utilisation of health services and, by extension, on health status? There is some evidence from the United States and Europe to suggest that they do. The Rand health insurance experiment is perhaps the most well-known analysis of the effect of user charges on the demand for ambulatory and secondary health care and health status. This randomised controlled trial took place during the 1970s and involved over 7,000 participants from six sites in the United States (Newhouse and The Insurance Experiment Group 1993). Its main findings were as follows (Brook *et al.* 1983; Lohr *et al.* 1986; Shapiro *et al.* 1986; Foxman *et al.* 1987; Lurie *et al.* 1987; Lurie *et al.* 1989):

- utilisation decreased as the level of cost-sharing through user charges increased
- increased cost-sharing had the same impact on the utilisation of effective and ineffective or medically inappropriate treatment
- although there were only small differences in health status between those receiving 'free' care and those subject to cost-sharing, cost-sharing appeared to affect people in low income groups and those in poor health dispropor-tionately; free care was beneficial to the health of these people

While the Rand experiment is widely regarded as a rigorous body of research, perhaps partly due to its unique experimental status, length and the expense involved), many have pointed to its weaknesses and limitations, and urged caution in the interpretation of its results. The main criticisms concern the study's generalisability, design issues such as the sample inclusion criteria,[10] the fact that there was an income-related ceiling on participants' out-of-pocket expenditure, the study's length, the range of health outcome measures used and the study's failure to take account of the fact that many decisions regarding utilisation are determined by providers rather than patients (Evans 1982; Relman 1983; van de Ven 1983; Schoenman 1993; Rice and Morrison 1994; Evans and Barer 1995).

Several European studies have analysed the impact of statutory co-payments on utilisation and health status. In the following sub-sections we summarise these studies, most of which are observational rather than experimental, and present evidence from Belgium, Denmark, Finland, France, Spain, Sweden and the United Kingdom.

The impact of user charges on utilisation of health services

UK studies consistently suggest that prescription charges may have some effect on patients' demand for drugs and their use of health services. Lavers (1989) analysed UK data from 1971 to 1982 and concluded that the use of prescription drugs was responsive to price, with an own-price elasticity of between –0.15 and –0.20.[11] Ryan and Birch (1991) found that increasing prescription charges was associated with a significant reduction in the use of prescribed drugs by patients who were not exempt from such charges between 1979 and 1985. O'Brien (1989) found that the own-price elasticity for prescription charges was –0.33 for the period 1969 to 1986. Own-price elasticities varied from a lower level of –0.23 between 1969 and 1977 to –0.64 between 1978 and 1986. Hughes and McGuire (1995) reassessed O'Brien's results, introducing two major changes to his econometric model, but found similar own-price elasticities.

Puig Junoy (1988) estimated an own-price elasticity of –0.13 for drug consumption in Spain between 1978 and 1985. However, other studies have found that during the same period about 30 to 40 per cent of prescriptions for retired individuals, who were exempt from drug co-payments, were in fact purchased on behalf of non-exempt family members (Lopez Bastida and Mossialos 2000). The relatively low sensitivity to price estimated by Puig Junoy may therefore be partly explained by the effect of substitution between different population groups.

Between 1988 and 1990 a deductible was applied to pharmaceuticals in Denmark, so that the consumption of prescription drugs below an annual maximum amount of DKK800 was no longer reimbursed by the statutory health care system. A national survey conducted in January 1990, combined with interviews at pharmacies in December 1989 and April 1990, found that 14 per cent of the population had exceeded the limit (Hansen *et al.* 1991). By the end of December 1989, 53 per cent of patients at pharmacies had exceeded the limit. More than 90 per cent of patients bought the prescribed drug, while fewer than 10 per cent asked their doctor to prescribe a cheaper drug. Overall, the introduction of the deductible reduced pharmaceutical consumption by only 2 to 3 per cent, but it was abolished at the beginning of 1991 in response to widespread public resistance (Christiansen *et al.* 1999).

The increase in cost-sharing for antibiotics introduced by the deductible had a significant impact on the prescribing patterns of general practitioners (GPs) in Denmark (Steffensen *et al.* 1997). A study carried out in North Jutland county showed that the increase in cost-sharing resulted in a decrease of 13 per cent in the consumption of antibiotics (measured in defined daily doses) between 1995 and 1996. The impact was high for broad-spectrum antibiotics (for example, the consumption of tetracyclines fell by 42 per cent), while the consumption of narrow-spectrum penicillins remained stable. It is not clear what effect the overall decline in consumption has had on health status. However, hospitals' use of antibiotics remained stable during the same period (Steffensen *et al.* 1997).

In Finland household contributions to health care funding increased and utilisation of certain health services declined following the economic recession and health care reforms of the early 1990s (Järvelin 2002). Between 1990 and 1994 user charges rose from 12.6 to 20.8 per cent of total expenditure on health care. During the same period user charges rose from 1.4 to 9.3 per cent of expenditure on outpatient care at health centres. The increases in private expenditure were distributed to the disadvantage of poorer people, who were more likely to make use of this type of care (Klavus 1997). A study to examine changes in the utilisation of doctors' services during the recession found that the total number of visits to a doctor declined by 16 per cent between 1991 and 1994 (Häkkinen *et al.* 1996). Most of this decline was due to fewer visits by chronically ill people. However, it is not clear whether the decline was caused by a fall in the supply of doctors or increases in user charges. Moderate user charges for accident and emergency services were introduced in 1991. An examination of the effect of these charges on rates of child hospitalisation for injuries showed that the overall rate of hospitalisation declined, but not statistically significantly, which suggests that the demand for care in paediatric injuries severe enough to require hospitalisation was not sensitive to charges (Ahlamaa-Tuompo 1999).

Research using Swedish data from the 1990s reveals the re-emergence of inequality in utilisation favouring richer people following major increases in user charges (Whitehead *et al.* 1997). A survey by the National Board of Health and Welfare found that about 8 per cent of all households who had a prescription in 1997 refrained from collecting drugs from the pharmacy at least once for financial reasons (National Board of Health and Welfare 1997). Another study shows that user charges present barriers for financially and psycho-socially disadvantaged groups in the Stockholm area; individuals who assessed their financial situation as being poor were ten times more likely to forgo health care than those who assessed their financial situation as being good (Elofsson *et al.* 1998). Researchers examining the effects of user charges on the use of prescription drugs among different socio-economic groups in Sweden found that higher user charges would result in a greater relative reduction in the consumption of 'discretionary' rather than 'essential' drugs (Lundberg *et al.* 1998). Individuals with poor health status are most price sensitive, but those most likely to reduce their consumption of prescription drugs are young people, the unemployed and those with poor health status, low levels of education or low incomes.

French research shows greater variation by socio-economic status in the use of doctor visits and pharmaceuticals than in the use of hospital care, which may be explained by the fact that hospital care is fully reimbursed by the statutory health care system, whereas the other types of care are not (Jourdain 2000).

Increases in statutory co-payments that do not affect the whole population have given rise to natural experiments in the European Union. A French study followed two groups of bank or insurance employees with employer-purchased complementary VHI after statutory co-payments were increased in 1994 (Chiappori *et al.* 1998). Most, but not all, insurers extended their coverage of statutory co-payments to compensate for the rise (increasing premiums at the same time). On average, individuals with extended coverage (the control group) experienced a decline in co-payments from 0.87 to 0.43 per cent, whereas individuals with coverage that was not extended (the treatment group) experienced a rise in co-payments from 0.95 to 10.2 per cent. The study found that the relative change in price did not have any impact on visits to GPs or specialists, but resulted in a modest reduction in GP home visits for patients in the treatment group. This suggests that the elasticity of demand for office visits may be close to zero for small variations in price due to the substantial transport and time costs that such visits may incur, so a 10 per cent increase in price will lead to a relatively small increase in total costs. In contrast, home visits are more likely to decline, because they are not associated with significant transport and time costs.

Two groups of researchers in Belgium were able to carry out a natural experiment following increases in co-payments in 1994, from which certain groups were exempt (Cockx and Brasseur 2001; van de Voorde *et al.* 2001). The general population and widowed, disabled, retired and orphaned individuals with incomes above a certain threshold experienced significant rises in co-payments for GP office visits (48 per cent), GP home visits (35 per cent) and specialist visits (60 per cent), while widowed, disabled, retired or orphaned individuals with incomes below the threshold were exempt from co-payments. The results of both studies resemble those of Chiappori *et al.* One study found average price elasticities of −0.13 for men and −0.03 for women (Cockx and Brasseur 2001). As in the French experiment, and in spite of a lower proportional increase in co-payments, the demand for GP home visits was most price elastic (−0.18 for men and −0.08 for women, compared to −0.06 and −0.01 respectively for GP office visits and −0.14 and −0.02 respectively for specialist visits). When compared to the control group (those exempt from co-payments), the demand for GP home visits decreased in the treatment group by 14 per cent for men and 9 per cent for women; the demand for GP office visits for women increased by 7 per cent, but the demand for other services did not change significantly. In contrast to Chiappori *et al,* the authors argue that the higher price elasticity for GP home visits is caused by the fact that home visits are a luxury, whereas GP visits and specialist visits by women are necessities. Overall, they found that the net efficiency gains arising from substantial increases in statutory co-payments were minimal. van de Voorde *et al.* found price elasticities for the general population of –0.39 to –0.28 for GP home visits, –0.16 to –0.12 for GP office visits and –0.10 for specialist visits, and lower and less significant elasticities for both groups of widowed, disabled, retired and orphaned individuals (van de Voorde *et al.* 2001). The authors were not able to calculate separate price elasticities for men and women.

The findings of these three studies should be treated with some caution. The authors only observed changes in utilisation over a short period[12] and the models they present fail to include important variables that affect the use of health services, such as income, health status and educational level (although Cockx and Brasseur did examine the effect of income and excluded high earners from the treatment group). Also, while the advantage of natural experiments lies in their ability to control for changes in other variables that may affect the group under study, their accuracy depends on the comparability of the control group to the treatment group (Besley and Case 2000). The average age of individuals in the French study's control group (38.9 years) was significantly lower than that of individuals in the treatment group (42.8 years), largely due to a higher proportion of individuals aged 65 and over (Chiappori *et al.* 1998). It is possible that the insurers that did not extend their coverage of statutory co-payments may have been concerned about over-utilisation of health services, in which case the study would have underestimated the impact of the co-payment on demand (Cockx and Brasseur 2001).

The impact of user charges on health status

The direct effect of user charges on health status is more difficult to measure, but a few studies provide some limited evidence. Theoretically, if the deterrent effect was directed at reducing the utilisation of so-called unnecessary services, then differential access to non-cost-effective services would not result in inequity in health status. However, there is some evidence to suggest that user charges deter the utilisation of cost-effective services and may therefore adversely affect health status.

After charges for eye tests were introduced in the United Kingdom, 19 per cent fewer patients were identified as requiring treatment or follow up for potentially blinding glaucoma (Laidlaw *et al.* 1994). As a result, such charges are likely to increase the prevalence of preventable blindness.

A Danish study found that the attendance rate at a preventive health examination for heart disease was 66 per cent when the service was provided free, but only 37 per cent when the service incurred a charge of US$40 (Christensen

1995a; Christensen 1995b). Attendees who paid for the examination showed a significantly lower level of risk of developing heart disease, and in particular a lower level of factors that could be known by the men themselves, such as smoking and being overweight. This suggests that those at higher risk of developing heart disease, and therefore more in need of preventive services, are those less likely to pay for them. Those who took part in the study agreed that heart disease was a serious condition that could be prevented by personal effort. The main reason for not taking part in the preventive health examination was the existence, or not, of a charge for the service.

Another Danish study examined the impact of user changes on influenza vaccination rates and found that charges are a barrier for many elderly patients and may prevent GPs from recommending vaccination to their older patients (Nexoe *et al.* 1997). Influenza vaccination is a cost-effective preventive measure in elderly patients, but user charges reduced the uptake of the vaccination in this population group.

Finnish studies of the effect of the introduction of a user charge for accident and emergency services found that the charge decreased visit rates by approximately 27 per cent for older children and 18 per cent for younger children, and that the decrease in visit rates was also pronounced in less painful conditions, leading the authors to conclude that the charge would have negligible long-term health consequences, given the magnitude and diagnosis-specificity of the reduction in demand (Ahlamaa-Tuompo *et al.* 1998a; Ahlamaa-Tuompo *et al.* 1998b).

Finally, an Irish study found that the use of accident and emergency services decreased with the introduction of a user charge (O'Grady *et al.* 1985). The user charge was also associated with reduced appropriate GP visits, which had adverse effects on blood pressure control and survival among high-risk patients.

Overall, the evidence regarding the impact of user charges on utilisation and health status in the European Union is limited. Nevertheless, the studies summarised in this section suggest that while user charges may reduce the utilisation of some health services, at least in the short term, they do not necessarily control expenditure growth in the long term. Furthermore, user charges appear to have a higher impact on people in lower socio-economic groups and may affect the health of poorer people. In spite of the absence of strong evidence, however, governments in some member states appear to find user charges an attractive policy option. In other member states, such as the United Kingdom, significant opposition to user charges has prevented the government from extending their use.

Voluntary health insurance and access to health care

An important distinction between statutory and voluntary health insurance in the European Union is that access to statutory health care depends on an individual's status as a citizen, resident or employee and is usually independent of ability to pay, whereas access to health care through VHI is almost always dependent on ability to pay. In practice, however, the extent to which the existence of VHI affects access to health care is partly determined by the characteristics of the statutory health care system. That is to say, if the statutory health care system guarantees all citizens equal access to health care for equal need (or, even better, equal utilisation for equal need), then access to VHI need not be an issue of concern, at least in terms of equity. Put another way, access to VHI may give rise to concerns about equity in so far as VHI is an individual's primary source of protection against the consequences of ill health. Broadly, therefore, the greater the role of VHI in providing access to effective health services that are a substitute for or complement to those provided by the state, the larger the impact it is likely to have on access to health care. Access to health care can also be affected where VHI plays a supplementary role, particularly if supplementary VHI provides faster access to treatment, but also if the boundaries between the public and the private sector are not clearly defined.

We suggest that there are three ways in which the existence of different types of VHI may present barriers to access. First, VHI may present a barrier to access where it is possible to purchase complementary VHI to cover the cost of user charges imposed by the statutory health care system, as is the case in several member states (Belgium, Denmark, France, Ireland, Italy, Luxembourg, Portugal and Sweden). It is both inequitable and inefficient for governments to establish a price mechanism in the health sector by introducing user charges, and then negate the effect of the mechanism for those who can afford to purchase complementary VHI.

The second way in which VHI may present a barrier to access is where it provides protection against the potentially catastrophic costs of ill health for individuals who are excluded from the statutory health care system or choose to opt out of it, as with substitutive VHI in the Netherlands and Germany. Due to the important role of substitutive VHI in providing social protection, the EU framework for regulating VHI allows the state to impose special conditions and regulatory controls on insurers providing substitutive VHI (European Commission 1992).[13] In recent years the Dutch and German governments have made substantial interventions in the market for substitutive VHI in order to ensure that older people, people with chronic illnesses and people on lower incomes have access to an adequate and affordable level of coverage (Mossialos and Thomson 2002b).

Third, VHI may present a barrier to access where it distorts or draws on public resources, to the detriment of public patients. This is most likely to happen when VHI does not operate independently of the statutory health care system; for example, if boundaries between public and private health care are not clearly defined, particularly if capacity is limited, if providers are paid by both the public and the private sector and if VHI creates incentives for health care professionals to treat public and private patients differently.

In the following sub-sections we examine these three scenarios with reference to complementary VHI and CMU in France, measures to ensure access to substitutive VHI in Germany and the Netherlands and equity concerns regarding the public/private divide in some member states offering supplementary VHI.

Complementary VHI and universal health coverage in France

There is some evidence to suggest that access to complementary VHI covering the cost of co-payments imposed in the statutory health care system is problematic for people with low incomes, particularly those who are just above the income threshold for any exemptions that may exist. Such individuals will be doubly disadvantaged in having to make co-payments in the first instance and then being unable to afford complementary VHI to cover the cost of these co-payments.

This type of complementary VHI is most prevalent in France, where it covered a third of the population in 1960, 50 per cent in 1970, 70 per cent in 1980 and 85 per cent in 1998 (Sandier et al. 2002). The likelihood both of being covered by complementary VHI and of having a high quality of coverage are largely dependent on income levels, employment status and age. Those who have little or no access to complementary VHI are much more likely to be from the lowest social classes (Bocognano et al. 2000). Employed and retired people are more likely to be covered than unemployed people, while employees and white-collar workers are more likely to be covered than unskilled workers (Mossialos and Thomson 2002b). A recent study shows that 59 per cent of unskilled workers have little or no VHI, compared to only 24 per cent of executives and professionals (Bocognano et al. 2000). Another study found that 94 per cent of individuals belonging to a household with an annual income of over €36,600 and 89 per cent of employees had complementary VHI, compared to only 65 per cent of those with less than €6,850 a year and 61 per cent of unemployed people (Blanpain and Pan Ké Shon 1997). The French system also appears to discriminate negatively against foreigners, young people aged between 20 and 24 and those over 70 years old, all of whom are less likely to be covered by complementary VHI. Furthermore, poorer people tend to have insurance cover of a lower quality than richer people, with 28 per cent of individuals earning over €36,600 a year judging their cover to be of good quality, compared to only 9 per cent of individuals with an annual household income under €6,850. This finding is strongly supported by Bocognano et al.'s study, which demonstrates that the level of coverage provided by complementary VHI increases significantly with income (Bocognano et al. 2000).

Research also shows that French people with complementary VHI consume more health care than those without (Breuil-Genier 2000), particularly ambulatory care, dental care and spectacles (Bocognano et al. 2000). Individuals with complementary VHI made 1.5 visits to a doctor in a three-month period, compared to 1.1 visits made by individuals without complementary VHI (Breuil-Genier 2000). On average they sought health care once every 73 days, compared to once every 100 days for those without complementary VHI.

In 1999, in order to address the inequalities in access to health care arising from unequal access to complementary VHI, the French government introduced a law on universal health coverage (CMU), extending complementary VHI coverage to people earning less than €550 per month who did not have any cover of this type (estimated on 31 December 2000 as 4.9 million people). Complementary VHI now covers about 94 per cent of the population (Sandier *et al.* 2002).

CMU benefits people on low incomes in two ways. First, since its introduction, the price of complementary VHI premiums in France is, in theory, no longer a barrier to access, except for people with incomes just above the threshold. Second, CMU requires insurers to provide CMU beneficiaries with benefits in kind rather than in cash. As a result, these low-income individuals are effectively exempt from making certain co-payments. Surveys reveal that the requirement to provide benefits in kind has increased equity in the French health care system (Mossialos and Thomson 2002b). That the introduction of CMU has increased access to outpatient care is reflected in the average outpatient per capita expenditure of CMU beneficiaries (€695) compared to people of the same age and sex insured in the main health insurance scheme (€538) (Girard and Merlière 2001). This suggests that the health status of CMU beneficiaries is low relative to other people. Unfortunately, there is also evidence to suggest that not everyone who should have benefited from CMU has done so, particularly those who have not had access to information about the scheme.

Access to substitutive VHI in Germany and the Netherlands

Although eligibility for substitutive VHI in Germany and the Netherlands depends on earning above a certain amount a year (the income threshold), there are individuals in both countries who find price an obstacle to obtaining an adequate level of substitutive VHI coverage. In the German context, where employees earning above an income threshold of €40,500 a year and their dependants can choose between the statutory health insurance scheme (*Gesetzliche Krankenversicherung* – GKV) and substitutive VHI, price is most likely to be problematic for older people, as substitutive VHI premiums tend to rise substantially with age and individuals aged over 55 are no longer permitted to return to the GKV, even if their incomes fall below the threshold.

High premium increases for older substitutive VHI policy holders put considerable pressure on the GKV in the early 1990s, as people would opt for substitutive VHI when they were young and then attempt to return to the GKV when their premiums became too expensive due to increasing age or ill health (Wasem 1995). In 1994 the German government took action to put a stop to this trend, announcing that the decision to opt for substitutive VHI would be irreversible for those aged 65 and over (Busse 2000). The recent Social Health Insurance Reform Act 2000 tightened the rules further by reducing the age limit for returning to the GKV to 54 (Comité Européen des Assurances 2000). In order to protect these people and ensure that they continue to be able to afford substitutive VHI cover, particularly if their incomes fall below the threshold, the government requires private health insurers to offer substitutive VHI policies at a standard rate (since 1994) to individuals aged 65 and over who have been voluntarily insured for a qualifying period of at least ten years, and (since 2000) at a standard rate for individuals aged 55 and over who have been voluntarily insured for at least ten years and whose incomes drop below the threshold.

Substitutive VHI policies sold at the standard rate provide benefits that match the benefits of the GKV and guarantee that premiums will not exceed the average maximum GKV contribution (or 1.5 times the contribution for married couples) (Comité Européen des Assurances 1997). However, as with all substitutive VHI policies, standard rate policies do not cover dependants, so even with the 50 per cent reduction for spouses, they are more expensive than the GKV, which covers dependants at no additional cost. To date, very few people have chosen standard rate policies, probably due to lack of information about eligibility. For this reason the 2000 Reform Act requires private health insurers to inform existing policy holders of the possibility of switching to another tariff category when their premiums go up and to advise policy holders aged 60 or over to switch to a standard rate policy or to switch to another tariff category that provides the same benefits for a lower premium. As a result of this change in the law, the numbers subscribing to the standard rate policy more than doubled between 1999 and 2000 (PKV 2001).

The 2000 Reform Act also tackled the problem of steeply rising premiums for older people by imposing a surcharge of up to 10 per cent of the gross premium on all new substitutive VHI policies and a premium increase of 2 per cent a year for five years for existing policy holders (Datamonitor 2000). By paying this surcharge, which goes into a shared reserve, policy holders can ensure that the cost of their premiums will not rise when they reach the age of 65.[14] New policy holders who choose not to pay the surcharge risk paying substantially increased premiums as they grow older. Finally, the 2000 Reform Act stipulates that private health insurers must inform potential substitutive VHI policy holders of the likelihood of increasing premiums, the possibility of limiting the increase in premiums with old age and the irreversibility of the decision to opt out of the GKV (Comité Européen des Assurances 2000).

There is some evidence to suggest that higher social classes in Germany use more specialist care than lower social classes, and it is claimed that this reflects their VHI coverage (Wysong and Abel 1990), although it may be linked to other personal determinants of access to health care, such as knowledge and educational levels.

In the Netherlands the government has also taken steps to ensure that people who are excluded from the statutory health insurance scheme for outpatient care and the first year of inpatient care (*Ziekenfondswet* – ZFW) are able to purchase an adequate level of substitutive VHI coverage for a fixed premium. The Dutch Health Insurance Access Act of 1986 (*Wet op de Toegang tot Ziektekostenverzekeringen* – WTZ) guarantees access to substitutive VHI for specific groups of people (Mossialos and Thomson 2002b). It was originally designed for individuals with substitutive VHI aged over 65 and younger self-employed people who had difficulty in purchasing substitutive VHI due to pre-existing conditions, but it now covers other groups, such as students whose parents are enrolled in the ZFW.

The WTZ Act enables the government to determine the level of benefits and the price of a fixed premium for a 'standard policy' that provides similar benefits to the ZFW (Mossialos and Thomson 2002b). However, the WTZ does not cover dependants, and therefore remains more expensive than the ZFW. Another essential difference between the ZFW and the WTZ is that the latter provides benefits in cash rather than in kind. Of all those excluded from the statutory health insurance scheme, 14.5 per cent are insured under the WTZ (4.2 per cent of the population). Because the fixed WTZ premium only covers half the cost of providing the standard policy, private health insurers receive full compensation from a central equalisation fund financed by an annual solidarity payment made by all those with substitutive VHI. This payment is currently fixed at €117.12 per year for children up to the age of 19 or €234.24 for individuals aged 20 to 64.

Equity concerns regarding supplementary VHI and the public/private divide

As we noted above, VHI could present a barrier to access in the statutory health care system by distorting the allocation of public resources, to the detriment of public patients. It is often argued that increasing VHI coverage reduces demand for statutory health services. However, the extent to which an expansion of VHI will result in lower demand for statutory health services depends on whether the boundary between the public and the private sector is clearly defined. In the United Kingdom, for example, where both sectors make use of the same supply of doctors, an increase in private sector activity per se may not lead to an increase in the public sector's capacity to tackle waiting lists. In fact, increasing private sector activity might actually reduce public sector capacity (see David Hughes' chapter on financial barriers to access in the United Kingdom).

An international study of the degree of horizontal equity achieved in health care utilisation in fourteen OECD countries (the United States, Canada and twelve EU member states, excluding Finland, France and Sweden) based on 1996 survey data found that after standardising for need differences across the income distribution, significant horizontal inequity in total doctor visits were only evident in Austria, Greece, Portugal and the United States (van Doorslaer et al. 2002).[15] However, when doctor visits were disaggregated into visits to GPs and visits to specialists, it was found that in every country except Luxembourg, richer people visited specialists more often than expected on the basis of need, while the use of GPs was relatively closely correlated with need, and in some countries was slightly pro-poor. 'Excess' specialist visits (those not correlated with need) by higher-income groups were particularly high in Ireland and Portugal. This is in contrast to an earlier study, based on older data, which did not find any significant inequity in specialist visits in Ireland or the United Kingdom (van Doorslaer et al. 2000). The more recent study also found that the degree and distribution of VHI coverage and regional disparities reduced equity in the use of doctor visits, although in most countries the negative effect on equity was fairly small (van Doorslaer et al.

2002).[16] However, the effect of VHI coverage on the use of specialist visits in Ireland was very high, indicating that the lack of VHI coverage does act as a barrier to specialist care for lower-income groups, in spite of their entitlement to free specialist care. VHI coverage also had a considerable impact on 'excess' specialist use in the United Kingdom, where supplementary VHI cover buys faster access to specialist care and, to a lesser extent, in Spain, Belgium, Denmark, Austria, Canada and Italy.

A Spanish study suggests that the existence of VHI may increase inequality in the Spanish health care system, with negative consequences for the health of poorer people (Borràs et al. 1999). The authors found that Catalonian women with supplementary VHI showed a higher percentage of cancer screening tests than the rest of the population, perhaps because double coverage by the Spanish National Health Service (NHS) and supplementary VHI provides women with more personalised care and increased involvement on the part of the physician. An investigation into inequalities by social class in access to and utilisation of health services in Catalonia found that although double coverage did not influence the social pattern of visits to health services provided by the NHS, there were social inequalities in the use of those health services provided only partially by the NHS (mostly dental care) and visits to a dentist were more frequent among those with complementary VHI (Rajmil et al. 2000).

Irish residents with supplementary/complementary VHI are able to make use of private and semi-private beds in public hospitals and publicly salaried consultants' private services in both public and private hospitals, in spite of long waiting times for public patients in public hospitals for certain types of specialist care. Private and semi-private beds have accounted for about 20 per cent of acute hospital beds since the process was introduced in the early 1990s (Nolan and Wiley 2000). The results of a recent study show that for each category of hospital admission, including planned (elective) care, emergency care and day care, utilisation by private patients has been increasing at a faster rate than utilisation by public patients (Wiley 2001). The study also found that private patients accounted for close to 30 per cent of discharges in 1999 and 2000, even though only about 20 per cent of acute beds at the national level are designated as private. Increasing use of public resources by private patients would appear to be at the expense of equity in the receipt of benefits in the overall health care system. Consequently, the Irish government's Health Strategy published in November 2001 proposed that all new beds made available in public hospitals will be solely for public use (Department of Health and Children 2001). The government also proposed to clarify the rules governing access to public beds, suggesting that action would be taken to suspend the admission of private patients for planned treatment if the maximum target waiting times for public patients were exceeded.

Finally, weak gate-keeping in the private sector in the Netherlands, leading to fewer GP contacts for VHI subscribers, has negatively affected gate-keeping in the public sector. Until recently it was compulsory for individuals with statutory health insurance to obtain a GP's referral before seeing a specialist or receiving treatment in hospital, but as a result of competition from voluntary health insurers, many of whom do not insist on referral, some statutory sickness funds have relaxed their gate-keeping requirements (Kulu-Glasgow *et al.* 1998).

Conclusions

Over the last twenty-five years, EU member states have extended statutory health insurance coverage to the whole – or almost the whole – population. At the same time, the comprehensiveness of statutory coverage has declined, partly due to the imposition of user charges and partly due to the exclusion of selected health services. This process of de-insurance is illustrated in Table 8.2, which shows how the proportion of private expenditure on health care increased, sometimes significantly, in many member states between 1975 and 1998.

In this chapter we have reviewed the effect of user charges for health services on utilisation and health status. A steady rise in the proportion of health care funded through out-of-pocket payments in many member states during the 1980s and 1990s suggests that governments have favoured the retention or introduction of user charges, in spite of the fact that the evidence regarding their impact is limited. Randomised controlled trials have not been carried out in Europe, and most studies in this area are observational, which is a major drawback. Nevertheless, there is sufficient evidence to suggest that user charges have a higher impact on the utilisation of people in lower socio-economic groups, although this impact has sometimes been short-lived. User charges may also affect the health of poorer people. While user charges do reduce the utilisation of some health services, at least in the short term, they do not necessarily control expenditure growth in the long term; supply-side policies may be more effective in containing health care costs.

The equity implications of any reduction in utilisation and consequent lowering of health status are likely to depend on the type of charge imposed and the exemption system in place. In this respect, deductibles may be more harmful than flat-rate fees or co-insurance, because poorer people may not be able to afford the initial financial outlay required. At the same time, co-insurance involves a greater degree of financial risk, as the cost of the treatment, and therefore the amount the user is required to pay, may not be known in advance.

More research needs to be done in this area, and future analysis should be based on individual rather than aggregate data. In the meantime, policy-makers debating whether or not to introduce user charges should give consideration to distributional issues, the design of exemption systems and the collection of appropriate data.

In this chapter we have also examined the extent to which VHI presents financial barriers to access in different EU member states. Our analysis suggests that VHI is likely to present financial barriers to access when it covers the cost of statutory co-payments, when it is the principal means of protection against the financial consequences of ill health, and when it distorts or draws on public resources to the detriment of public patients. As the French experience of complementary VHI demonstrates, it is neither equitable nor efficient for governments to establish a price mechanism in the health sector by introducing user charges, and then negate the effect of the mechanism for those who can afford to purchase VHI. The EU regulatory framework for VHI only allows governments to intervene in substitutive VHI markets, and both the German and the Dutch governments have introduced substantial regulation to ensure that elderly, chronically ill or poorer people have access to an affordable level of substitutive VHI cover. Finally, some governments have found that the existence of VHI can reduce access for publicly funded patients, and are taking steps to clarify the boundaries between public and private health care.

There is a general need for greater scrutiny of VHI markets in the European Union, as current levels of data availability are insufficient for evidence-based policy-making. If policy-makers are to be persuaded that the EU regulatory framework works to the advantage of consumers, they must have access to better information about how these markets operate (and in whose interest). More specifically, research should focus on the potential for different types of VHI to present financial barriers to access, particularly where policy-makers are considering an expansion of VHI markets.

Acknowledgements

We would like to thank Anna Dixon for her comments on an earlier draft of this chapter. Any errors remain the responsibility of the authors.

Notes

1 The European Union is currently made up of fifteen member states. Established by Belgium, France, Germany, Italy, Luxembourg and the Netherlands in 1950, the founding members were subsequently joined by Denmark, Ireland and the United Kingdom (in 1973), Greece (in 1981), Spain and Portugal (in 1986) and Austria, Finland and Sweden (in 1995). In 2000, per capita GDP ranged from US$16,058 in Greece to US$24,135 in the United Kingdom to US$28,354 in Denmark (in purchasing power parities). Average per capita GDP was US$25,427.

2 We define VHI as health insurance that is taken up and paid for at the discretion of individuals or employers on behalf of individuals. VHI can be offered by public or quasi-public bodies and by for-profit (commercial) and non-profit private organisations. VHI can be classified according to whether it substitutes for cover that would otherwise be available from the state (substitutive VHI), provides complementary cover for services excluded or not fully covered by the state, including cover for user charges imposed by the statutory health care system (complementary VHI), or provides supplementary cover for faster access and increased consumer choice (supplementary VHI) (Mossialos and Thomson 2002a).

3 Self-employed people in Belgium are only covered for 'major risks' such as inpatient care. Coverage of 'minor risks' (visits to a general practitioner or specialist, drugs, nursing care, most types of physiotherapy, dental care and minor surgical procedures) can be obtained by purchasing substitutive VHI.

4 Self-employed people, civil servants and their dependants make up the remainder. Most self-employed people are excluded from the statutory health insurance scheme. The government directly reimburses a significant proportion of civil servants' health care expenditure.

5 In 1999 85 per cent of the French population was covered by complementary VHI to cover the cost of statutory co-payments, while 28.9 per cent of the Dutch population is excluded from statutory coverage of primary care and acute inpatient care.

6 In a regressive funding system the poor spend a greater proportion of their income on health care than the rich; in a proportionate funding system everybody spends the same proportion; in a progressive funding system the rich spend a greater proportion than the poor.

7 Here, essential is defined in terms of disease category and in the light of judgments about effectiveness.

8 Unequal treatment for equal need.

9 Elasticity of demand is a measurement of the change in demand for a good or service caused by a) a change in the price of that good or service (own-price elasticity), b) a change in the price of another good or service (cross-price elasticity) or c) a change in the income of the person demanding the good or service (income elasticity).

10 People aged over 62 and those too disabled to work were excluded from the study.

11 That is, a 1 per cent increase in the price of the prescription drug led to a reduction of between 0.15 and 0.20 per cent in the quantity purchased.

12 Chiappori *et al.* and Cockx and Brasseur observed changes over a one-year period. Van de Voorde *et al.* studied data over a ten-year period (1986 to 1995), but only two of those years were after the 1994 rise in co-payments.

13 The EU regulatory framework is based on the third non-life insurance directive issued by the European Commission in 1992, which created a single market for VHI in the European Union and abolished national controls on the price of VHI premiums and prior notification of policy conditions. Regulation can only be justified if it is in the interest of 'the general good'.

14 Premium rises were largely caused by inaccurate premium calculations and inadequate ageing reserves. Substitutive VHI in Germany is written in the same way as life insurance. Premiums are loaded to reflect the age at which an individual purchases a policy. In theory, therefore, premiums should not rise as policy holders age. However, during the 1990s premiums rose steeply as people aged, because insurers had based their premium calculations on average life expectancy, failing to account for the longer than average life expectancy enjoyed by substitutive VHI policy holders, who tend to come from higher socio-economic groups.

15 In this context, horizontal equity is defined as the degree to which visits to a doctor are distributed according to need. As the European data used in the study were obtained from the third wave of the European Community Household Panel, the authors' estimates of need are based on self-reported health status.

16 As the authors note, however, the data they used did not provide any information regarding households' or individuals' liability for co-payments.

References

Abel-Smith, B. (1994) *An Introduction to Health: Policy, Planning and Financing*. London: Longman.

Ahlamaa-Tuompo, J. (1999) 'The effect of user charges and socio-demographic environment on paediatric trauma hospitalisation in Helsinki in 1989–1994', *European Journal of Epidemiology*, 15(2): 133–9.

Ahlamaa-Tuompo, J., Linna, M. and Kekomaki, M. (1998a) 'Impact of user charges and socio-economic environment on visits to paediatric trauma unit in Finland', *Scandinavian Journal for Social Medicine*, 26(4): 265–9.

Ahlamaa-Tuompo, J., Linna, M. and Kekomaki, M. (1998b) 'User charges and the demand for acute paediatric traumatology services', *Public Health*, 112(5): 327–9.

Andersen, R.M. (1995) 'Revisiting the behavioral model and access to medical care: does it matter?', *Journal for Health Social Behaviour*, 36(1): 1–10.

Besley, T. and Case, A. (2000) 'Unnatural experiments? Estimating the incidence of endogenous policies', *The Economic Journal*, 110(467): 672–94.

Blanpain, N. and J.-L. Pan Ké Shon (1997) 'L'assurance complémentaire maladie: une diffusion encore inégale', *INSEE Première*, 523 (June).

Bocognano, A., Couffinhal, A., Dumesnil, S. and Grignon, M. (2000) *Which Coverage for Whom? Equity of Access to Health Insurance in France*. Paris: CREDES.

Borràs, J., Guillen, M., Sánchez, V., Juncá, S. and Vicente, R. (1999) 'Educational level, voluntary private health insurance and opportunistic cancer screening among women in Catalonia (Spain)', *European Journal of Cancer Prevention*, 8:427–34.

Breuil-Genier, P. (2000) 'Généraliste puis spécialiste: un parcours peu fréquent', *INSEE Première*, 709, April.

Brook, R.H., Ware, J.E., Rogers, W.H., Keeler, E.B., Davies, A.R., Donald, C.A., Goldberg, G.B., Lohr, K.N., Masthay, P.C. and Newhouse, J.P. (1983) 'Does free care improve adults' health? Results from a randomized controlled trial', *New England Journal of Medicine*, 309(23): 1426–34.

Busse, R. (1999) 'Cost containment in Germany: twenty years' experience'. In E. Mossialos and J. Le Grand (eds) *Health Care and Cost Containment in the European Union*. Aldershot: Ashgate.

Busse, R. (2000) *Health Care Systems in Transition: Germany*. Copenhagen: European Observatory on Health Care Systems.

Busse, R. (2001) 'Risk structure compensation in Germany's statutory health insurance', *European Journal of Public Health*, 11(2): 174–7.

Chalkley, M. and Robinson, R. (1997) *Theory and Evidence on Cost Sharing in Health Care: An Economic Perspective*. London: Office of Health Economics.

Chiappori, P.A., Durand, F. and Geoffard, P.Y. (1998) 'Moral hazard and the demand for physician services: first lessons from a French natural experiment', *European Economic Review*, 42(3–5): 499–511.

Christensen, B. (1995a) 'Characteristics of attenders and non-attenders at health examinations for ischaemic heart disease in general practice', *Scand J Prim Health Care*, 13(1): 26–31.

Christensen, B. (1995b) 'Payment and attendance at general practice preventive health examinations', *Family Medicine*, 27(8): 531–4.

Christensen, J.K., Pedersen, L.L. and Hvenegaard, A. (1999) *The Nature and Impact of Danish Health Care Reforms (1988–1999)*. Final country report for 'EU market forces'. Copenhagen: Danish Institute for Health Services Research and Development.

Christiansen, T., Enemark, U., Clausen, J. and Poulsen, P. (1999) 'Health care and cost containment in Denmark'. In E. Mossialos and J. Le Grand (eds) *Health Care and Cost Containment in the European Union*. Aldershot: Ashgate.

Cockx, B. and Brasseur, C. (2001) *The Demand for Physician Services: Evidence from a Natural Experiment*. Louvain-la-Neuve: Catholic University of Louvain.

Comité Européen des Assurances (1997) *Health Insurance in Europe 1997*. Paris: CEA.

Comité Européen des Assurances (2000) *Health Insurance in Europe: 1998 data, CEA ECO 12 (July 2000)*. Paris: CEA.

Creese, A. (1997) 'User fees: they don't reduce costs and they increase inequity [editorial]', *British Medical Journal*, 315(7102): 202–3.

Datamonitor (2000) *European Health Insurance 2000: What's the Prognosis, Doctor?* London: Datamonitor.

Department of Health and Children (2001) *Quality and Fairness: A Health System for You, The Department of Health and Children's Health Strategy 2001*. Dublin: Department of Health and Children.

Diderichsen, F., Varde, V. and Whitehead, M. (1997) 'Resource allocation to health authorities: the quest for an equitable formula in Britain and Sweden', *British Medical Journal*, 315: 875–8.

Elofsson, S., Unden, A.L. and Krakau, I. (1998) 'Patient charges – a hindrance to financially and psychosocially disadvantaged groups seeking care', *Social Science Medicine*, 46(10): 1375–80.

European Commission (1992) 'Council Directive 92/49/EEC of 18 June 1992 on the coordination of laws, regulations and administrative provisions relating to direct insurance other than life assurance and amending Directives 73/239/EEC and 88/357/EEC (third non-life insurance Directive)', *OJEC* L 228(11 August 1992): 1–23.

European Commission (1999) *A Concerted Strategy for Modernising Social Protection*, COM(99)347 final. Brussels: European Commission.

European Commission (2001) *Healthcare: Commission Proposes Three Common EU Objectives for Healthcare and Care for the Elderly – Access for All, High Quality, Financial Sustainability*. Brussels: European Commission.

Evans, R.G. (1982) 'Health care in Canada: patterns of funding and regulation'. In G. McLachlan and A. Maynard (eds) *The Public Private Mix for Health*. London: Nuffield Provincial Hospitals Trust.

Evans, R.G. and Barer, M.L. (1995) 'User fees for health care: why a bad idea keeps coming back (or, what's health got to do with it?)', *Canadian Journal on Aging*, 14(2): 360–90.

Eversley, J. and Webster, C. (1997) 'NHS charges. Light on the charge brigade', *Health Services Journal*, 107(5562): 26–8.

Fallberg, L.H. (2000a) 'Patients' rights in Europe: where do we stand and where do we go?', *European Journal of Health Law*, 7: 1–3.

Fallberg, L.H. (2000b) 'Patients' rights in the Nordic countries', *European Journal of Health Law*, 7: 123–43.

Foxman, B., Valdez, R.B., Lohr, K.N., Goldberg, G.A., Newhouse, J.P. and Brook, R.H. (1987) 'The effect of cost sharing on the use of antibiotics in ambulatory care: results from a population-based randomized controlled trial', *J Chronic Dis*, 40(5): 429–37.

Girard, I. and Merlière, J. (2001) 'La consommation de soins de ville des bénéficiaires de la CMU au terme d'une année de remboursements', *Point STAT*, 31(March): 1–8.

Glennerster, H., Hills, J., Travers, T. and Hendry, R. (2000) *Paying for Health, Education and Housing: How Does the Centre Pull the Purse Strings?* Oxford: Oxford University Press.

Gulliford, M.C., Morgan, M., Hughes, D., Beech, R., Figueroa-Muñoz, J.L., Gibson, B., Hudson, M., Arumugam, C., Connell, O., Mohiddin, A. and Sedgwick, J. (2001) *Access to Health Care: A Scoping Exercise*. London: NHS R&D Service Delivery and Organisation Programme.

Häkkinen, U. (1999) 'Cost containment in Finnish health care'. In E. Mossialos and J. Le Grand (eds) *Health Care and Cost Containment in the European Union*. Aldershot: Ashgate.

Häkkinen, U., Rosenqvist, G. and Aro, S. (1996) 'Economic depression and the use of physician services in Finland', *Health Economics*, 5(5): 421–34.

Hanning, M. (1996) 'Maximum waiting time guarantee: an attempt to reduce waiting times in Sweden', *Health Policy*, 36(1): 17–35.

Hanning, M. and Spångberg, U.W. (2000) 'Maximum waiting time – a threat to clinical freedom? Implementation of a policy to reduce waiting times', *Health Policy*, 52: 15–32.

Hansen, H., Jensen, C.H. and Rasmussen, N.K. (1991) 'The distribution effects of the Danish 800 crown rule. Preliminary results of the DIKE study. Choice of drugs and drugs used by the population', *Ugeskr Laeger*, 153(20): 1413–15.

Harrison, A. (2000) 'The war on waiting', *Health Care UK*, Winter: 52–60.

Hjortsberg, C. and Ghatnekar, O. (2001) *Health Care Systems in Transition: Sweden.* Copenhagen: European Observatory on Health Care Systems.

Hughes, D. and McGuire, A. (1995) 'Patient charges and the utilisation of NHS prescription medicines: some estimates using a cointegration procedure', *Health Economics*, 4(3): 213–20.

Järvelin, J. (2002) *Health Care Systems in Transition: Finland.* Copenhagen: European Observatory on Health Care Systems.

Jourdain, A. (2000) 'Equity of a health system' *European Journal of Public Health*, 10(2): 138–142.

Kasper, J. D. (2000) 'Health-care utilization and barriers to health care'. In G.L. Albrecht, R. Fitzpatrick and S.C. Scrimshaw (eds) *Handbook of Social Studies in Health and Medicine.* London: Sage Publications.

Klavus, J. (1997) 'User fees and fee policy in health care'. In M. Heikkilä and H. Uusitalo (eds) *The Cost of Cuts. Studies on Cutbacks in Social Security and Their Effects in the Finland of the 1990s.* Helsinki: STAKES (National Research and Development Centre for Welfare and Health).

Kulu-Glasgow, I., Delnoij, D. and de Bakker, D. (1998) 'Self-referral in a gatekeeping system: patients' reasons for skipping the general practitioner', *Health Policy*, 45: 221–3.

Kutzin, J. (1998) 'The appropriate role for patient cost sharing'. In R.B. Saltman, J. Figueras and C. Sakellarides (eds) *Critical Challenges for Health Care Reform in Europe.* Buckingham: Open University Press.

Laidlaw, D., Bloom, O., Hughes, A.O., Sparrow, J.M. and Marmion, V.J. (1994) 'The sight test fee: effect on ophthalmology referrals and rate of glaucoma detection', *British Medical Journal*, 309: 634–6.

Lamata, F. (1995) *El copago en la financiación de los servicios sanitarios públicos* [Co-payment in the financing of public health care services]. *Modelos de coparticipación del usuario en la financiación de la sanidad pública* [Proposals of joint participation of users in the financing of the public health care system]. Madrid: Fundación de Ciencias de la Salud.

Lavers, R.J. (1989) 'Prescription charges, the demand for prescriptions and morbidity', *Applied Economics*, 21(8): 1043–52.

Lohr, K.N., Brook, R.H., Kamberg, C.J., Goldberg, G.A., Leibowitz, A., Keesey, J., Reboussin, D. and Newhouse, J.P. (1986) 'Effect of cost sharing on use of medically effective and less effective care', *Medical Care*, 24(9 supplement): S31–38.

Lopez Bastida, J. and Mossialos, E. (2000) 'Pharmaceutical expenditure in Spain: cost and control', *International Journal of Health Services*, 30(3): 597–616.

Lundberg, L., Johannesson, M., Isacson, D.G.L. and Borgquist, L. (1998) 'Effects of user charges on the use of prescription medicines in different socio-economic groups', *Health Policy*, 44(2): 123–34.

Lurie, N., Kamberg, C.J., Brook, R.H., Keeler, E.B. and Newhouse, J.P. (1989) 'How free care improved vision in the health insurance experiment', *American Journal of Public Health*, 79(5): 640–2.

Lurie, N., Manning, W.G., Peterson, C., Goldberg, G.A., Phelps, C.A. and Lillard, L. (1987) 'Preventive care: do we practice what we preach?', *American Journal of Public Health*, 77(7): 801–4.

Ministry of Health and Social Affairs (2002) *International Forum on Common Access to Health Care Services*. Stockholm: Ministry of Health and Social Affairs.

Ministry of Health Welfare and Sport (2000) Personal communication with the Ministry's Public Information Office.

Ministry of Health Welfare and Sport (2002) *Health Insurance in the Netherlands: Status as of 1 January 2002*. The Hague: Ministry of Health, Welfare and Sport.

Mossialos, E. and Le Grand, J. (1999) 'Cost containment in the EU: an overview'. In E. Mossialos and J. Le Grand (eds) *Health Care and Cost Containment in the European Union*. Aldershot: Ashgate.

Mossialos, E. and Thomson, S. (2002a) 'Voluntary health insurance in the European Union: a critical assessment', *International Journal of Health Services*, 32(1): 19–88.

Mossialos, E. and Thomson, S. (2002b) *Voluntary Health Insurance in the European Union*. Report prepared for the Directorate General for Employment and Social Affairs of the European Commission. Available online at: http://europa.eu.int/comm/employment_social/soc-prot/social/index_en.htm. London: London School of Economics and Political Science.

National Board of Health and Welfare (1997) *Can Households Afford Medicine?* Results from a survey conducted in October 1997. Stockholm: National Board of Health and Welfare.

Newhouse, J.P. and The Insurance Experiment Group (1993) *Free for all? Lessons from the RAND Health Insurance Experiment*. Cambridge and London: Harvard University Press.

Newton, J.N., Henderson, J. and Goldacre, M. (1995) 'Waiting list dynamics and the impact of earmarked funding', *Briish Medical Journal*, 311: 783–5.

Nexoe, J., Kragstrup, J. and Ronne, T. (1997) 'Impact of postal invitations and user fee on influenza vaccination rates among the elderly. A randomized controlled trial in general practice', *Scandinavian Journal of Primary Health Care*, 15(2): 109–12.

Nolan, B. and Wiley, M.M. (2000) *Private Practice in Irish Public Hospitals*. Dublin: Oak Tree Press in association with the Economic and Social Research Institute.

Noyce, P.R., Huttin, C., Atella, V., Brenner, G., Haaijer-Ruskamp, F.M., Hedvall, M. and Mechtler, R. (2000) 'The cost of prescription medicines to patients', *Health Policy*, 52(2): 129–45.

O'Brien, B. (1989) 'The effect of patient charges on the utilisation of prescription medicines', *Journal of Health Economics*, 8(1): 109–32.

O'Grady, K.F., Manning, W.G., Newhouse, J.P. and Brook, R.H. (1985) 'The impact of cost sharing on emergency department use', *New England Journal of Medicine*, 313(8): 484–90.

Okma, K. and Poelert, J.D. (2001) 'Implementing prospective budgeting for Dutch sickness funds', *European Journal of Public Health*, 11: 178–81.

Organisation for Economic Co-operation and Development (2001) *Health Data 2001*. Paris: Organisation for Economic Co-operation and Development.

Pereira, J., Campos, A.C., Ramos, F., Simões, J. and Reis, V. (1999) 'Health care reform and cost containment in Portugal'. In E. Mossialos and J. Le Grand (eds) *Health Care and Cost Containment in the European Union*. Aldershot: Ashgate.

Persson, A. and Guzelgun, Z. (1998) 'Taxes, premiums, user charges: financing from the point of view of consumers', *Dev Health Econ Public Policy*, 7: 255–72.

PKV (2001) *Private Health Insurance: Facts and Figures 2000/2001*. Available online at: http://www.pkv.de/default.asp. Köln: Verband der privaten Krankenversicherung e.V.

Puig Junoy, J. (1988) 'Gasto farmaceutico en Espana: effectos de la participacion del usuario en el coste', *Investigaciones Economicas*, 12(1): 45–68.

Rajmil, L., Borrell, C., Starfield, B., Fernandez, E., Serra, V., Schiaffino, A. and Segura, A. (2000) 'The quality of care and influence of double health care coverage in Catalonia (Spain)', *Arch Dis Child*, 83(3): 211–14.

Relman, A. (1983) 'The Rand health insurance study: is cost sharing dangerous to your health? [editorial]', *New England Journal of Medicine*, 309(23): 1453.

Rice, N. and Smith, P.C. (2002) 'Strategic resource allocation and funding decisions'. In E. Mossialos, A. Dixon, J. Figueras and J. Kutzin (eds) *Funding Health Care: Options for Europe*. Buckingham: Open University Press.

Rice, T. and Morrison, K.R. (1994) 'Patient cost sharing for medical services: a review of the literature and implications for health care reform', *Medical Care Review*, 51(3): 235–87.

Robinson, R. (2002) 'User charges for health care'. In E. Mossialos, A. Dixon, J. Figueras and J. Kutzin (eds) *Funding Health Care: Options for Europe*. Buckingham: Open University Press.

Ryan, M. and Birch, S. (1991) 'Charging for health care: evidence on the utilisation of NHS prescribed drugs', *Social Science Medicine*, 33(6): 681–7.

Sandier, S., Polton, D., Paris, V. and Thomson, S. (2002) 'France'. In A. Dixon and E. Mossialos (eds) *Health Care Systems in Eight Countries: Trends and Challenges*. Report commissioned by the Health Trends Review, HM Treasury. London: European Observatory on Health Care Systems.

Schoenman, J.A. (1993) *Use of Patient Cost Sharing as a Means of Controlling Health Care Costs*. HOPE/Western Consortium Conference on Health Reforms in Central Europe. Prague: National Strategies for Cost Containment.

Shapiro, M.F., Ware, J.E. and Sherbourne, C.D. (1986) 'Effects of cost sharing on seeking care for serious and minor symptoms. Results of a randomized controlled trial', *Ann Intern Med*, 104(2): 246–51.

Sissouras, A., A. Karokis and E. Mossialos (1999) 'Health care and cost containment in Greece'. In E. Mossialos and J. Le Grand (eds) *Health Care and Cost Containment in the European Union*. Aldershot: Ashgate.

Steffensen, F.H., Schonheyder, H.C., Tolboll Mortensen, J., Nielsen, K. and Toft Sorensen, H. (1997) 'Changes in reimbursement policy for antibiotics and prescribing patterns in general practice', *Clin Microbiol Infect*, 3(6): 653–7.

Towse, A. (1999) 'Could charging patients fill the cash gap in Europe's health care systems?', *Eurohealth*, 5(3): 27–9.

van de Ven, W.P. (1983) 'Effects of cost-sharing in health care', *Effective Health Care*, 1(1): 47–56.

van de Voorde, C., van Doorslaer, E. and Schokkaert, E. (2001) 'Effects of cost sharing on physician utilization under favourable conditions for supplier-induced demand', *Health Economics*, 10(5): 457–71.

van Doorslaer, E., Koolman, X. and Puffer, F. (2002) 'Equity in the use of physician visits in OECD countries: has equal treatment for equal need been achieved?'. In P. Smith (ed.) *Measuring Up: Improving Health System Performance in OECD Countries*. Paris: Organisation for Economic Co-operation and Development.

van Doorslaer, E., Wagstaff, A., van der Burg, H., Christiansen, T., De Graeve, D., Duchesne, I., Gerdtham, U.G., Gerfin, M., Geurts, J., Gross, L., Hakkinen, U., John, J., Klavus, J., Leu, R.E., Nolan, B., O'Donnell, O., Propper, C., Puffer, F., Schellhorn, M., Sundberg, G. and Winkelhake, O. (2000) 'Equity in the delivery of health care in Europe and the US', *Journal of Health Economics*, 19(5): 553–83.

Wagstaff, A., van Doorslaer, E., Calonge, S., Christiansen, T., Gerfin, M., Gottschalk, P., Janssen, R., Lachaud, C., Leu, R.E., Nolan, B. *et al.* (1992) 'Equity in the finance of health care: some international comparisons', *Journal of Health Economics*, 11(4): 361–87.

Wagstaff, A., van Doorslaer, E., van der Burg, H., Calonge, S., Christiansen, T., Citoni, C., Gerdtham, U.G., Gerfin, M., Gross, L., Hakinnen, U., Johnson, P., John, J., Klavus, J., Lachaud, C., Lauritsen, J., Leu, R., Nolan, B., Peran, E., Pereira, J., Propper, C., Puffer, F., Rochaix, L., Rodríguez, M., Schellhorn, M., Sundberg, G. and Winkelhake, O. (1999) 'Equity in the finance of health care: some further international comparisons', *Journal of Health Economics*, 18(3): 263–90.

Wasem, J. (1995) 'Regulating private health insurance markets'. In K. Okma (ed.) *Four Country Conference on Health Care Reforms and Health Care Policies in the United States, Canada, Germany and the Netherlands*. Amsterdam, 23–25 February 1995. Amsterdam: Ministry of Health, Welfare and Sport.

Whitehead, M., Evandrou, M., Haglund, B. and Diderichsen, F. (1997) 'As the health divide widens in Sweden and Britain, what's happening to access to care?', *British Medical Journal*, 315: 1006–9.

Wiley, M.M. (2001) 'Reform and renewal of the Irish health care system: policy and practice'. In *Budget Perspectives: Proceeding of a Conference held on 9 October 2001*. Dublin: The Economic and Social Research Institute.

Willman, J. (1998) *A Better State of Health*. London: Profile Books Ltd/The Social Market Foundation.

World Health Organization (2000a) '43 European countries have yet to enact laws on patients' rights', press release EURO 07/00. Copenhagen: WHO Regional Office for Europe.

World Health Organization (2000b) Patients' rights and citizens' empowerment: through visions to reality, Joint consultation between the WHO Regional Office for Europe, the Nordic Council of Ministers and the Nordic School of Public Health, Copenhagen, 22–23 April 1999. Copenhagen: WHO Regional Office for Europe.

Wysong, J.A. and Abel, T. (1990) 'Universal health insurance and high-risk groups in West Germany: implications for US health policy', *The Milbank Quarterly*, 68(4): 527–60.

Chapter 9

Access to dental services

Barry Gibson

Introduction

Dental disease is chronic and has an almost universal impact. It is not directly life threatening and tends to be readily normalised. Delays in the uptake of dental care are common, leading to the conclusion that there is a significant symptom iceberg in dentistry (Locker 1988b). The most recent estimates suggest that around two million people in England have unmet dental needs (Department of Health 2000).

Access in dentistry implies not only utilisation but also whether a person's utilisation conforms to the underlying professional norm that regular access to dental services should be maintained. Dental utilisation and access in oral health services research is therefore defined in relation to whether or not access has occurred within a set time period, usually over the previous one to two years. However, survey data suggest that the concept of 'routine attendance' is of questionable value (Tickle and Worthington 1992; Nuttall and Davies 1991; Murray 1996). Significant proportions of people only attend the dentist when they are in pain but traditional measures of dental utilisation often do not distinguish between preventive and illness behaviours.

The traditional approach to access in oral health services research has uncovered many factors that influence patterns of routine and non-routine attendance at the dentist. This chapter will provide a brief summary of the more recent findings. It will also examine issues of access to fluoridation which is considered a public health measure of choice and could be used to reduce inequalities in dental health.

Availability of dental services

A major recent feature in UK dental provision, especially in south east England, has been a shift away from National Health Service (NHS) dentistry towards private dental provision. The number of dentists working in the general dental service has increased, but the amount of time they spend treating NHS patients has decreased. This has led to problems accessing NHS dentistry, and the NHS dental service has been described as 'patchy and unreliable' (Department of Health 2000: 13). There are a number of reasons for problems in the availability of dental services, some of which are related to the dental contract while others relate to workforce issues.

The NHS dental contract was changed in 1991, with the aim of developing a process of continuing care for patients. The result was that access to dental services depended on the maintenance of patients' registration. Up to 40 per cent of the population in England in 1998 did not attend the dentist on a regular basis (Kelly *et al.* 2000). When a patient's registration lapses there is the possibility that their dentist may not accept them back for treatment. Some 40 per cent of dental practices are not currently accepting children or adults for registration for continuing care (Audit Commission 2002). The result is that people may find it increasingly difficult to access NHS dental treatment (Department of Health 2000). They may find themselves in the position of receiving only emergency treatments which are included in the 'occasional' treatments list. This is a restricted list of treatments which are provided to people who are not registered. These treatments are temporary in nature and for the relief of pain only; they include temporary restorations as opposed to more permanent restorations.

Changes in the contract for NHS general dental services also required dentists to provide 24-hour emergency cover for all patients registered at their practices. Demand for recalled (emergency) dental services increased dramatically and there was a 234 per cent increase in the associated costs between 1990 and 1993 (Crawford 1993). These increasing costs were described as unreasonable, and centralised services were then developed (Gibbons and West 1996). In turn the demand for centralised emergency dental services increased by 51 per cent between 1989 and 1995 (Dickinson and Guest 1996). Significant numbers of patients now use these services as a routine form of dental care (Thomas *et al.* 1997) but treatment at these services is characterised by dental extractions and prescriptions of analgesics. Increasing numbers of people attending these services are self referred and not registered with a general dental practitioner (Thomas *et al.* 1997). It remains unclear if this pattern is a result of differences in treatment provision or of differing patient needs. Some dentists have argued that the expansion of the use of emergency dental services is an indicator that patients are now using emergency dental services for primary dental care (Rhodes 1990).

Only about 500 (3 per cent) of dentists in England perform no work for the NHS, but the amount of time most dentists spend on NHS work has decreased. In 1993, 75 per cent of dentists said they received at least three-quarters of their earnings from the NHS, but by 1999 this figure had decreased to 58 per cent (Department of Health 2000). In deciding to provide private dental care, dental practitioners appear to be trading off conflicts of professional identity. They want to provide a service to the highest standards of care, with the latest technology, alongside preventive and caring delivery (Calnan *et al.* 2000). The NHS fee-per-item system does not encourage preventive dentistry, and dentists perceive that they are given perverse incentives. Significant regional variations in basic underlying costs (such as accommodation) have also led to varying pressures on dentists to organise around the provision of private dental treatment. Conflicting personal and professional values appear to have both facilitated and impeded this tendency. These in turn may have led to major regional variations in the accessibility of NHS dentistry (Calnan *et al.* 2000). In short it is felt that the NHS provides a piecemeal system and that it makes sense for dentists to attend to more than one 'paymaster' (Calnan *et al.* 2000; Sintonen and Maljanen 1995).

A significant change in the dental workforce is that over 52 per cent of new graduates from dental schools moving into this traditionally male-dominated profession are now women. Women dentists are more likely to prefer to work in salaried practices, in the community dental services or in paediatric dentistry. They work more flexible hours and take longer career breaks (Newton *et al.* 2000a). If more women are working part time there is a likelihood that there will be a shortage of dental personnel and in addition the preference of women for salaried employment means that remuneration patterns may have to change to fit their demands (Department of Health 2000). Other workforce issues concern the impact of the emerging 'Professions Complementary to Dentistry' (PCDs) including dental nurses, hygienists and therapists. There is also increasing specialisation of professional roles with the potential emergence of more high street specialist oral surgeons, orthodontists and periodontists. This represents a move away from highly centralised secondary services to more diverse services. These developments may have significant implications in terms of access to primary and secondary care respectively (Department of Health 2000).

Personal characteristics and utilisation of dental services

Different age groups vary in their utilisation of dental services. Early access to dental services has been shown to be important in the prevention and early detection of dental disease in children. However, the Child Dental Health Survey in the United Kingdom demonstrated a strong association between the attendance patterns of mothers and children (O'Brien 1994). Dentists recommend the use of fluoride supplements in combination with professionally delivered forms of prevention such as fissure sealants (Stewart *et al.* 1999). In one study only 15 per cent of children aged six to 17 years had received dental sealants whilst 73 per cent had attended the dentist in the past twelve months. More white children whose parents had higher income levels and at least one year of undergraduate education had sealants (24 per cent) than similar socio-economic status black children (11 per cent). Additionally 'black' children whose parents had a college education were less likely to have dental visits during the past 12 months (68 per cent) than white children of similar socio-economic status (86 per cent). Trends in dental service utilisation by adolescents show increasing numbers of adolescents attending (88 per cent in 1977 to 95 per cent in 1995) the dentist in the last year (Honkala *et al.* 1997). However, dental attendance consistently declined from the age of 11 to 18 years in the period between 1977 and 1995 irrespective of gender.

The UK Adult Dental Health Survey found in 1998 that among adults with teeth, twice as many reported attending the dentist on a regular basis as those who reported only attending for pain (30 per cent). The proportion of dentate adults reporting going to the dentist on a regular basis in the UK appeared to have increased over the preceding ten years, from 43 per cent to 59 per cent (Kelly *et al.* 2000). It has been found that as people age, while their visits to the doctor increase, their visits to the dentist decrease (Ettinger 1992). Considerable research has been conducted with respect to older people since they appear to be one of the groups least likely to attend the dentist despite having most to gain from dental care (Watt and Sheiham 1999). Despite consistently low levels of utilisation it has emerged that there are often high levels of need for treatment in these age groups (Locker *et al.* 1991; Marino 1994). This combination of findings has led to the conclusion that the inverse care law exists in relation to dental utilisation for older people (Dolan and Atchison 1993; Locker *et al.* 1991). Traditional predictors of utilisation of general health services such as functional dependence, infrequent physician contact, and perceived barriers have shown little value in predicting dental service utilisation. Rather it was found that dentate status, perceived need and recent symptom experiences were the best predictors of service utilisation (Holtzman *et al.* 1990).

The importance of dentate status in predicting access to dental services is now well established (Ettinger 1992; Dolan and Atchison 1993; Warren *et al.* 2000). Locker *et al.* (1991) determined that 90.1 per cent of dentate compared with 53.4 per cent of edentulous people sought care when they perceived they needed it. In the previous year almost three quarters of dentate people had made a visit whereas less than two fifths of edentulous people had done so (Locker *et al.* 1991). Lundgren *et al.* (1995) found that 91 per cent of people with teeth in Sweden had visited the dentist in the last year whereas only 32 per cent without teeth had done so. Perceived need for care has therefore been significantly associated with dental utilisation (Atchison *et al.* 1993). It is also argued that age is not a factor in dental attendance especially when samples are stratified by dentate status (Locker *et al.* 1991). UK data would tend to support this claim with dentate adults between the ages of 55 to 74 years being more likely to attend the dentist on a regular basis than younger dentate adults (Kelly *et al.* 2000).

The relationship between gender and the utilisation of dental services follows a similar relationship with access to other health services. Data from the Adult Dental Health Survey indicates that women (66 per cent) are significantly more likely than men (52 per cent) to report seeking regular check-ups. This data also suggests that women who are employed full time are less likely to report attending the dentist on a regular basis (63 per cent) than women employed part time (71 per cent). Women who are unemployed on the other hand are least likely to report attending for regular dental checks (54 per cent) and young adult males are the group least likely to seek dental care (Honkala *et al.* 1997; Kelly *et al.* 2000).

People with chronic disability are said to have poorer oral health, higher untreated disease levels and more extractions than their healthy peers (Wilson

1992). There is some indication that there are significant barriers in the availability and accessibility of dental services for various groups of disabled patients.

Zimmerman *et al.* (1995) reporting on Swedish data determined that 38 per cent of migrants had visited a dentist and 41 per cent of these had visited the dentist only once since migration. The average gap between arrival in Sweden and attendance at the dentist was 4.5 years (Zimmerman *et al.* 1995). Locker *et al.* (1998) found that Canadian-born subjects were more likely (72.6 per cent) than immigrant adolescents (42.8 per cent) to report visiting for regular dental care. Canadian-born adolescents were also more likely (81.7 per cent) to report accessing services within the last 12 months than those of migrant status (61.3 per cent).

In the UK there are significant inequities in relation to dental utilisation. People from manual social classes are less likely to attend the dentist on a regular basis (49 per cent) than those in non-manual social classes (65 per cent). This is despite the fact that those people in manual occupational groups have more decayed and unsound teeth than those from non-manual groups (Kelly *et al.* 2000). These differences in dental status only exist in relation to those younger than 45 years; above this age the differences seem to disappear (Kelly *et al.* 2000).

Inequalities in adults are generally less marked than those in children (Watt and Sheiham 1999). In the UK among toddlers of one to four years, 40 per cent from manual social classes had decay experience compared with 16 per cent of those from non-manual social classes. In the Child Dental Health Survey data between the ages of five to 15 years, the only variable strongly and independently associated with the number of decayed and/or filled primary teeth was the pattern of the child's dental attendance (Watt and Sheiham 1999; O'Brien 1994). Finally, for both 12- and 15-year-olds there was an association between social class and decay (Watt and Sheiham 1999). Despite these findings it is reported that together these social characteristics explained only 8 per cent of the variance in the level of known decay in the primary dentition and only 7 per cent and 8 per cent respectively of the variation of decay experience in permanent dentition (Watt and Sheiham 1999; O'Brien 1994). In addition to this there remain significant regional variations in decay experience throughout the UK, with children in the north-east region experiencing much more decay than the UK average (Watt and Sheiham 1999).

Much of the work demonstrating a relationship between ethnic group and utilisation has been conducted in the US. This has shown that ethnic minority groups utilise dental care less than whites (Andersen and Davidson 1997). In 1989, 4.7 per cent of Americans had never visited a dentist. The proportions of people who had never had a dental visit was higher for blacks 6.9 per cent, Hispanics 12.6 per cent and Mexican Americans 17.2 per cent (Bolden *et al.* 1993). Oral health status data in the US indicate consistently that ethnic minorities have more unmet need. It is further proposed that cost and the availability of dental insurance or public programmes are factors that contribute to differential access for low-income groups and minorities (Bolden *et al.* 1993) (see Chapter 7).

Multi-factorial models and utilisation dental services

Many though not all of the descriptive studies outlined above are based on emerging relationships within a particular empirical perspective. Common problems in studies of dental utilisation include non-probability sampling and a lack of focus on low-income and minority groups (Manski and Magder 1998). In order to address some of these shortcomings Manski and Magder (1998) examined the relationship between dental care utilisation and several socio-economic variables including employment status, dental insurance coverage, sex, health status, education, age and race. Their data were extracted from a nationally representative US data set using and constructing a set of explanatory variables (Manski and Magder 1998). All of the following predictors had a significant relationship with accessing the dentist in the last year: age, income, sex, race, marital and dental insurance status. The odds ratio of blacks attending the dentist was 0.66 times that of whites whilst controlling for all other predictors. The odds ratio for Hispanics reporting a dental visit was 0.80 (Manski and Magder 1998). A limitation of this work is the lack of information on the reason why the person attended the dentist in the last year. This leads to the possibility of confusion between health and illness utilisation (Locker *et al.* 1991).

Other work has attempted to explain access in terms of either social disadvantage (Dolan and Atchison 1993), personality factors (Kennedy *et al.* 1990) or by highlighting barriers to and delays in access. One of the few qualitative studies to evaluate barriers to dental care, and one which is widely cited in the UK, is the work of Finch and colleagues (1989). This study reported on focus group data and highlighted that anxiety and cost were the two major barriers to the receipt of dental care. Other barriers identified by participants included the impersonal nature of the dental encounter, white coats, bright lights, the conveyor belt approach to dental treatment, and fear of being reprimanded and being treated as though they were a mouth (Finch *et al.* 1989).

Several multi-factorial models have been applied in attempts to explain access to dental services. The Expanded Social Behavioural Model of Andersen (Andersen and Davidson 1997) formed the basis of the International Collaborative Study on Oral Health Outcomes (ICS-II) in 11 different countries. The Expanded Social Behavioural Model is a useful sensitising model which helps draw together diverse independently related variables to help predict dental utilisation (Davidson and Andersen 1997), preventive behaviour (Davidson *et al.* 1997) and to a lesser extent oral health outcomes (Marcus *et al.* 1997) for diverse ethnic and age groups. In terms of dental utilisation it appears that regardless of ethnic group membership, the likelihood of dental utilisation was higher if people were not edentulous, had a usual source of dental care, and had experienced oral pain or discomfort. In this model no predisposing oral health beliefs maintained predictive power regardless of ethnic group. Of significant interest however is that the explanatory power of the model appeared to be considerably lower for Baltimore African-Americans

($r^2 = 0.288$), San Antonio Hispanics ($r^2 = 0.313$), Lakota Native Americans ($r^2 = 0.175$), Navajo Native Americans ($r^2 = 0.137$) versus San Antonio white persons ($r^2 = 0.421$) and Baltimore white adults ($r^2 = 0.424$). This finding calls into question the cross-cultural power of the model to explain dental utilisation patterns. It may also however reflect difficulties in the selection of predisposing factors, enabling resources and the perception of need for dental treatment which carry the same meaning for diverse ethnic groups.

Financial and organisational barriers to utilisation

In the NHS, patients are required to contribute co-payments for dental treatment services amounting to 80 per cent of the cost of care (Audit Commission 2002). However, some groups are exempt, including children and young people under 18, young people in full time education, pregnant women and new mothers. Older people do not automatically have exemption from NHS dental charges; exemption is only available to older people on low incomes. People on Income Support and their partners are entitled to exemption from NHS dental charges.

As dental services are not usually free at the point of delivery, patients generally want to know more about what the dentist is going to do, why, and how much it is going to cost. Particular attention to these factors in the UK Adult Dental Health Survey indicates that these concerns appear to increase between the ages of 16 and 34 years when most people are beginning to experience out-of-pocket restorative dental treatment for the first time (Kelly et al. 2000). Additionally it has been reported that more people are negotiating to pay for dental treatment over a period of time rather than at the point of delivery (Kelly et al. 2000). Even though cost has been demonstrated as one of the traditional barriers to dental treatment, the increasing importance of private dental services means that such a view of costs may no longer be appropriate (Hancock et al. 1999). A recent Finnish study suggested that the time taken to get to a dental practice was a more significant determinant of access than the fee per treatment (which had a small but significant effect) (Sintonen and Maljanen 1995).

The relative importance of time and costs probably differs by socio-economic group. The cost of dental treatment impacts disproportionately on those who have the highest level of need (Kelly et al. 2000), therefore it is important to account for differences between the direct and indirect costs associated with treatment. Conversely, if financial barriers are removed through exemption from charges, or through insurance, then providers may be more able to induce demand for more complex treatments. UK data show that patients who are exempt from dental charges tend to receive more expensive treatments under the NHS. In the period between April 1999 and March 2000 in England and Wales the average costs of treatment for those not receiving benefits was £34.78 whereas the average costs for those in receipt of benefits was £51.10 (Dental Practice Board 2000b). Those in receipt of benefits tended to receive more complicated treatments such as crowns and bridges (Dental Practice Board 2000a).

The nature of the relationship between private and public dental care has not yet been adequately analysed. The 1998 Adult Dental Health Survey confirmed that many more people said their last course of dental treatment was provided by the private sector (18 per cent compared with 6 per cent in 1988) and this difference was even more marked in the south of England (24 per cent compared with 6 per cent in 1988). These changes were noted most particularly in those from non-manual backgrounds (Stephens 2000) and among those who reported attending for regular check-ups (4 per cent to 19 per cent) (Kelly *et al.* 2000). There is a need for research into the underlying dynamics of this shift especially with respect to access. Little is currently known about how people decide to attend for private dental treatment and there is little data available on the processes involved in attending the dentist (Gibson *et al.* 2000).

Utilisation of dental services – policy developments

It is clear that current patterns of supply and use of dental services are unsatisfactory. Major concerns relate to the geographical accessibility of services, the nature of the financial incentives to dentists, the financial barriers to patients, and other aspects of patients' help-seeking behaviours. Recent policy documents have suggested that these problems should be addressed through a combination of increased investment, redesign and modernisation of existing services, and the development of new services (Department of Health 2000; Department of Health 2002) (see also Chapter 5). The overall aim of these developments is to provide, and promote, universal access to NHS dentistry in the UK.

In the NHS Dental Plan the government proposed to improve the availability of NHS dental care by allocating funds to improve the remuneration of dentists working for the NHS. Additional funds were allocated for improvements to dental practices (Department of Health 2000). More recent proposals have suggested that a range of updated methods of remunerating dentists should be piloted by different commissioning primary care trusts. These include options for salaried status, and use of capitation fees and practice allowances, in addition to revised fee-for-service schedules. Under these proposals patients will be offered oral health assessments focused on the prevention of disease, and treatments will be performed according to agreed evidence-based protocols. These reforms aim to reduce the current direct association between dentists' remuneration and the type of treatment offered (Department of Health 2002). The NHS Direct telephone helpline is now being used to advise callers on how they can access NHS dentists. Finally, a number of special dental access centres are being set up in order to provide dental care to people who are not otherwise registered with a dentist (Department of Health 2000).

Oral health outcomes

Oral health services should be evaluated in terms of outcomes as well as processes (Dolan 1995; Buck and Newton 2001). In the UK, oral health has improved in the last 30 to 40 years but considerable inequalities persist (Department of Health 2000). Since the late 1960s, the greatest improvements in oral health have occurred in children where disease levels have declined over 50 per cent in five-year-olds and 75 per cent in 12- to 15-year-olds respectively. The percentages of adults with no teeth have fallen dramatically since the late1960s (from 37 per cent in 1968 to 12 per cent in 1998) (Department of Health 2000). The likelihood is that because older adults are retaining their teeth longer they are less likely to need dentures but more likely to already have crowns and large fillings which will in turn require maintenance.

The measurement of oral-health-related outcomes is multidimensional involving oral health status, oral-health-related quality of life measures and satisfactory access to dental services (Atchison and Andersen 2000). The International Collaborative Study on Oral Health Outcomes provides an opportunity to investigate this wider range of indicators in diverse populations. Atchison and Andersen (2000) report finding that older adults in Baltimore were doing well in terms of tooth loss, perceived oral health, physical and social functioning, and moderately high with respect to periodontal status and satisfaction with access to dental services. In contrast Native Americans (comprising Navajo from New Mexico, Chinle from Arizona and Lakota from South Dakota) have poor outcomes in terms of tooth loss, periodontal status, and consumer satisfaction, and moderate with respect to perceived oral health and physical and social functioning (Atchison and Andersen 2000). The conclusions of this work indicated that significant inequalities existed in oral health outcomes.

The traditional approach to the problem of access to dental services has focused on individuals and the 'factors' that affect their utilisation of dental health care. However, dental services only accounted for 28, 43 and 34 per cent of the variance in the disease status of 5- to 12-year-olds in the UK in 1985, 1987 and 1989 respectively. Social factors including the presence or not of fluoridated toothpaste has accounted for 53, 62 and 57 per cent of the variance over the same time period (Nadanovsky and Sheiham 1994). International comparisons have yielded similar results, although these data are subject to uncertainty due to missing data, differing diagnostic criteria and treatment patterns (Nadanovsky and Sheiham 1995). The implications are that a multi-sectoral approach to oral health promotion should be adopted. The range of interventions suggested to reduce inequalities include community development programmes, re-orientating health services according to need (making equity targets explicit), oral health education, the development of healthy policies and the creation of healthy environments including healthy schools and fluoridation (Watt and Sheiham 1999).

Access to fluoridated water supplies

Fluoridation can adjust the conditions of the environment in such a way as to provide significant oral health gain for whole populations (Hinman *et al.* 1996; Kelman 1996; Lennon 2000). Fluoridation has been proposed as a public health measure that can reduce inequalities in oral health for school children (McNally and Downie 2000). The evidence to support this claim is nevertheless disputed (Cohen and Locker 2001; Diesendorf 1995; Hawkins *et al.* 2000).

The most influential work to date on the issue of evidence concerning the benefits of water fluoridation is the systematic review conducted by the NHS Centre for Reviews and Dissemination in York (Freudenberg 2000; McDonagh *et al.* 2000b). This review found that while there appeared to be consistent benefits accruing from fluoridation, in terms of the prevention of oral disease, the quality of the evidence was low to moderate. The review also indicated that fluoridation did not reduce inequalities as much as had originally been claimed (McDonagh *et al.* 2000a; McDonagh *et al.* 2000b) and stressed that the benefits of water fluoridation should be considered carefully together with the risks. Risks related to evidence of fluorosis (mottled teeth) in communities and the concentration of fluoride in drinking water. They were unable to find an association between water fluoridation and any other adverse health effect. The York review concluded that health care professionals needed to consider carefully the negative effects of fluorosis (Department of Health 2000; McDonagh *et al.* 2000b). The consideration of risk, however, is a highly charged problem in society and it is well established in sociology that risk claims tend to multiply (Luhmann 1993). Water fluoridation has been no exception. Some of the negative effects claimed for fluoridation range from fluorosis (mottled teeth), cancer, osteoporosis, and Alzheimer's disease amongst others (Groves 2001; Isaacson *et al.* 1997; Weeks *et al.* 1993; Yiamouyiannis 1983).

Early sociological attempts to explain the fluoridation controversy uncritically accepted that the scientific evidence for fluoridation was strongly supportive. The result was an assumption that the measure was itself logical and those who opposed the measure were in some way alienated or misinformed (Martin 1989). The decision not to provide access to fluoridation is not necessarily irrational; the pro-fluoridationists' claims are better interpreted, not as statements of incontrovertible fact based on the rationality of science, but as part of a strategy to promote fluoridation (Martin 1989). The following are the summary arguments proposed by Martin (1989):

Pro-fluoridationist argument:

> The evidence for the benefits of fluoridation is quite substantial, while the evidence for harm is limited and dubious. I think the likely benefits outweigh the possible dangers, hence I support fluoridation because it is the cheapest and easiest way to make sure every child reaps the benefits.
>
> (Martin 1989: 66)

The anti-fluoridationist argument

> Though the evidence for the benefits of fluoridation is quite substantial there is some doubt about it. Since fluoridation is not necessary for good teeth, we should forgo the benefits if there is some slight cause of harm. Some scientists claim that a small percentage of the population could be harmed by fluoride. Therefore I oppose fluoridation of water supplies and favour the voluntary use of fluoride tablets by those who want to take them.
>
> (Martin 1989: 66)

From this perspective the fluoridation controversy is not a matter of fact but a matter of values in relation to the evaluation of risks and benefits. This position has recently been adopted by some in dentistry (Cohen and Locker 2001). The prospects for the provision of access to fluoridated water supplies seem poor, although instances do exist where successful public relations campaigns have been fought (Castle 1987). Such instances serve to illustrate the social and political nature of the debate.

Conclusions

Oral disease has a widespread distribution in most Western populations and a significant symptom iceberg has been identified (Locker 1988b). Access to personal dental services is important because oral disease can cause significant morbidity and in some instances severe disablement (Locker 1988a). Most research in dentistry concerning questions of access has focused on individual utilisation of personal dental services. This research has been largely quantitative and descriptive and has produced a relatively long list of associations between personal and service characteristics and access to dental services. Whilst these provide some insights into the influences on access to dental services, much more is required in order to explain the mix of health and illness behaviours. Other approaches adopted in the dental literature have used the multi factorial Social Behavioural and Health Belief models with relative success. Yet as indicated earlier in this book (see Chapter 4) these models fail to take into account patient's perspectives on the access to dental care. Research perspectives influenced by the interpretive paradigm are relatively underdeveloped in dentistry and it follows that there have been few attempts to apply such approaches to the analysis of access to dental services (Finch *et al.* 1989; Gibson *et al.* 2000).

Within oral health services research, the importance of questions of access to personal dental services remains contested since it has been shown that social factors have accounted for more of the variance in dental disease levels in the populations of many Western societies (Nadanovsky and Sheiham 1994; Nadanovsky and Sheiham 1995). It has been argued that fluoridation of the water supplies should be considered another oral health service which would be of greater merit to whole populations than current individual dental services.

References

Andersen, R.M. and Davidson, P.L. (1997) 'Ethnicity, aging, and oral health outcomes: a conceptual framework', *Advances in Dental Research*, 11: 203–9.

Atchison, K.A. and Andersen, R.M. (2000) 'Demonstrating successful ageing using the International Collaborative Study for Oral Health Outcomes', *Journal of Public Health Dentistry*, 60: 282–8.

Atchison, K.A., Mayer-Oakes, S.A., Schweitzer, S.O., Lubben, J.E., De Jong, F.J. and Matthias, R.E. (1993) 'The relationship between dental utilization and preventive participation among a well-elderly sample', *Journal of Public Health Dentistry*, 53: 88–95.

Audit Commission (2002) *Dentistry. Primary Dental Care Services in England and Wales*. London: Audit Commission.

Bolden, A.J., Henry, J.L. and Allukian, M. (1993) 'Implications of access, utilization and need for oral health care by low income groups and minorities on the dental delivery system', *Journal of Dental Education*, 57: 888–900.

Buck, D. and Newton, T. (2001) 'Non-clinical outcome measures in dentistry: publishing trends 1988–98', *Community Dentistry and Oral Epidemiology*, 29: 2–8.

Calnan, M., Silvester, S., Manley, G. and Taylor-Gooby, P. (2000) 'Doing business in the NHS: exploring dentists' decisions to practise in the public and private sectors', *Sociology of Health and Illness*, 22: 742–64.

Castle, P. (1987) *The Politics of Fluoridation: The Campaign for Fluoridation in the West Midlands of England*. London: John Libbey and Company Limited.

Cohen, H. and Locker, D. (2001) 'The science and ethics of water fluoridation', *Journal of the Canadian Dental Association*, 67: 578–80.

Crawford, A.N. (1993) 'Guest leader: emergency dental services', *British Dental Journal*, 174: 84.

Davidson, P.L. and Andersen, R.M. (1997) 'Determinants of dental care utilization for diverse ethnic and age groups', *Advances in Dental Research*, 11: 254–62.

Davidson, P.L., Rams, T.E. and Andersen, R.M. (1997) 'Socio-behavioural determinants of oral hygiene practices among USA ethnic and age groups', *Advances in Dental Research*, 11: 245–53.

Dental Practice Board (2000a) *Dental Treatments: GDS Annual Statistics*. Eastbourne: Dental Practice Board Data Services Branch.

Dental Practice Board (2000b) *Gross Fees: General Dental Services Annual Statistics*. Eastbourne: Dental Practice Board Data Services Branch.

Department of Health (2000) *Modernising NHS Dentistry – Implementing the NHS plan*, London: Department of Health.

Department of Health (2002) *NHS Dentistry: Options for Change*. London: Department of Health.

Dickinson, T. M. and Guest, P. G. (1996) 'An audit of demand and provision of emergency dental treatment', *British Dental Journal*, 181: 86–7.

Diesendorf, M. (1995) 'How science can illuminate ethical debates – A case-study on water fluoridation', *Fluoride*, 28: 87–104.

Dolan T.A. (1995) 'Research issues related to optimal oral health outcomes', *Medical Care*, 33: 106–22.

Dolan, T.A. and Atchison, K.A. (1993) 'Implications of access, utilization and need for oral health care by the non-institutionalized and institutionalized elderly on the dental delivery system', *Journal of Dental Education*, 57: 876–87.

Ettinger, R.L. (1992) 'Attitudes and values concerning oral health and utilisation of services among the elderly', *International Dental Journal*, 42: 373–84.

Finch, H., Keegan, J., Ward, K. and Sen., S.S. (1989) *Barriers to the Receipt of Dental Care: A Qualitative Research Study*. London: British Dental Association.

Freudenberg, N. (2000) 'Health promotion in the city: a review of current practice and future prospects in the United States', *Annual Review of Public Health*, 21: 473–503.

Gibbons, D.E. and West, B.J. (1996) 'Dentaline: an out of hours emergency dental service in Kent', *British Dental Journal*, 180: 63–6.

Gibson, B.J., Drennan, J., Hanna, S. and Freeman, R. (2000) 'An exploratory qualitative study examining the social and psychological processes involved in regular dental attendance', *Journal of Public Health Dentistry*, 60: 5–11.

Gift, H.C., Andersen, R.M. and Chen, M.-S. (1997) 'The principles or organization and models of delivery of oral health care'. In Pine, C.M. (ed.) *Community Oral Health*, Chapter 16. Oxford: Wright.

Groves, B. (2001) *Fluoride: Drinking Ourselves to Death?* Dublin: Newleaf.

Hancock, M., Calnan, M. and Manley, G. (1999) 'Private or NHS general dental service care in the United Kingdom? A study of public perceptions and experiences', *Journal of Public Health Medicine*, 21: 415–20.

Hawkins R.J., Leaje J.L. and Adegbembo, A.O. (2000) 'Water fluoridation and the prevention of dental caries', *Journal of the Canadian Dental Association*, 66: 620–3.

Hinman, A.R., Sterritt, G.R. and Reeves, T.G. (1996) 'The U.S. experience with fluoridation', *Community Dental Health*, 13: 5–9.

Holtzman, J.M., Berkey, A.B. and Mann, J. (1990) 'Predicting utilization of dental services by the aged', *Journal of Public Health Dentistry*, 50: 164–71.

Honkala, E., Kuusela, S., Rimpela, A., Rimpela, M. and Jokela, J. (1997) 'Dental services utilization between 1977 and 1995 by Finnish adolescents of different socioeconomic levels', *Community Dentistry and Oral Epidemiology*, 25: 385–90.

Isaacson, R.L., Varner, J.A. and Jensen, K.F. (1997) 'Toxin-induced blood vessel inclusions caused by the chronic administration of aluminium and sodium fluoride and their implications for dementia. Neuro protective agents', *Annals of the New York Academy of Science*, 825: 152–66.

Kelly, M., Steele, J., Nuttall, N., Bradnock, G., Morris, J., Nunn, J., Pine, C., Pitts, N., Treasure, E. and White, D. (2000) *Adult Dental Health Survey: Oral Health in the United Kingdom, 1998*. London: The Stationery Office.

Kelman, A.M. (1996) 'Fluoridation – the Israel experience', *Community Dental Health*, 13: 42–6.

Kennedy, B.D., Aldwin, C.M., Bosse, R., Douglass, C.W. and Chauncey, H.H. (1990) 'Personality and dental care utilization: findings from the VA longitudinal study', *Special Care in Dentistry*, 10: 102–6.

Lennon, M.A. (2000) 'Water fluoridation: a test of the government's public health credentials', *Community Dental Health*, 17: 210–11.

Locker, D. (1988a) 'Measuring oral health: a conceptual framework', *Community Dental Health*, 5: 3–18.

Locker, D. (1988b) 'The symptom iceberg in dentistry: treatment-seeking in relation to oral and facial pain', *The Journal of the Canadian Dental Association*, 54: 271–4.

Locker, D., Clarke, M. and Murray, H. (1998) 'Oral health status of Canadian-born and immigrant adolescents in North York, Ontario', *Community Dentistry Oral Epidemiology*, 26(3): 177–81.

Locker, D., Leake, J.L., Lee, J., Main, P.A., Hicks, T. and Hamilton, M. (1991) 'Utilization of dental services by older adults in four Ontario communities', *Journal of Canadian Dental Association (Journal de l'Association Dentaire Canadienne)*, 57: 879–86.

Luhmann, N. (1993) *Risk: A Sociological Theory*. New York: Aldine De Gruyter.

Lundgren, M., Osterberg, T., Emilson, G. and Steen, B. (1995) 'Oral complaints and utilization of dental services in relation to general health factors in a 88-year-old Swedish population', *Gerodontology*, 12: 81–8.

Manski, R.J. and Magder, L.S. (1998) 'Demographic and socioeconomic predictors of dental care utilization', *Journal of the American Dental Association*, 129: 195–200.

Marcus, M., Reifel, N. and Nakazono, T.T. (1997) 'Clinical measures and treatment needs', *Advances in Dental Research*, 11: 263–71.

Marino, R. (1994) 'Oral health of the elderly: reality, myth, and perspective', *Bulletin of the Pan American Health Organization*, 28: 202–10.

Martin, B. (1989) 'The sociology of the fluoridation controversy: a re-examination', *The Sociological Quarterly*, 30: 59–76.

Martin, B. (1999) 'Fluoridation: the left behind?', *Arena*, 89: 32–8.

McDonagh, M.S., Whiting, P.F., Wilson, P.M., Sutton, A.J., Chestnutt, I., Cooper, J., Misso, K., Bradley, M., Treasure, E. and Kleijnen, J. (2000a) *NHD CRD. A Systematic Review of Public Water Fluoridation*. York: University of York (Report 18), York Centre for Reviews and Dissemination.

McDonagh, M.S., Whiting, P.F., Wilson, P.M., Sutton, A.J., Chestnutt, I., Cooper, J., Misso, K., Bradley, M., Treasure, E. and Kleijnen, J. (2000b) 'Systematic review of water fluoridation', *British Medical Journal*, 321: 855–9.

McNally M. and Downie J. (2000) 'The ethics of water fluoridation', *Journal of the Canadian Dental Association*, 66: 592–3.

Murray, J. (1996) 'Attendance patterns and oral health', *British Dental Journal*, 181: 339–42.

Nadanovsky, P. and Sheiham, A. (1994), 'The relative contribution of dental services to the changes and geographical variations in caries status of 5- and 12-year-old children in England and Wales in the 1980s', *Community Dental Health*, 11: 215–23.

Nadanovsky, P. and Sheiham, A. (1995) 'Relative contribution of dental services to the changes in caries levels of 12-year-old children in 18 industrailized countries in the 1970's and early 1980's', *Community Dentistry and Oral Epidemiology*, 23: 331–9.

Newton, J.T.N., Kavanagh, D., Gibbons, D.E. and Zoitopolous, L. (2000a) *The London Primary Care Studies Programme, Local Primary Care Research Priority Exercise, Primary Care Research Priorities – Dentistry (Lambeth, Southwark and Lewisham, Bromley)*. London: London Regional Research and Development RDC01862.

Newton, J.T.N., Thorogood, N. and Gibbons, D.E. (2000b) 'The work patterns of male and female dental practitioners in the United Kingdom', *International Dental Journal*, 50: 61–8.

Nuttall, N.M. and Davies, J.A. (1991) 'The frequency of dental attendance of Scottish dentate adults between 1978 and 1988', *British Dental Journal*, 171:161–5.

O'Brien, M. (1994) *Children's dental health in the United Kingdom 1993*. London: Office of Population Censuses and Surveys.

Rhodes, F.J. (1990) 'Analysis of patterns of use of an emergency dental service', *British Dental Journal*, 169: 99–100.

Sintonen, H. and Maljanen, T. (1995) 'Explaining the utilisation of dental care. Experiences from the Finnish dental market', *Health Economics*, 4: 453–66.

Slade, G.D. (ed.) (1997) *Measuring Oral Health and Quality of Life*. Proceedings of a conference held 13–14 June 1996, at the University of North Carolina-Chapel Hill. Chapel Hill: University of North Carolina.

Stephens, C. (2000) 'Using expert systems and ISDN support to improve the delivery of orthodontic advice in primary care', NRR Project: N0500035821; Funding organisation name: NHS Executive North West.

Stewart, D.C., Ortega, A.N., Alos, V., Martin, B., Dowshen, S.A. and Katz, S. H. (1999) 'Utilization of dental services and preventive oral health behaviors among preschool-aged children from Delaware', *Pediatric Dentistry*, 21: 403–7.

Thomas, T.W., Satterthwaite, J., Absi, E.G. and Shepherd, J.P. (1997) 'Trends in the referral and treatment of new patients at a free emergency dental clinic since 1989', *British Dental Journal*, 182: 11–14.

Tickle, M. and Worthington, H.V. (1992) 'Factors influencing perceived treatment need and the dental attendance patterns of older adults', *British Dental Journal*, 182: 96–100.

Warren, J.J., Cowen, H.J., Watkins, C.M., and Hand, J.S. (2000) 'Dental caries prevalence and dental care utilization among the very old', *Journal of the American Dental Association*, 131: 1571–9.

Watt, R. and Sheiham, A. (1999) 'Inequalities in oral health: a review of the evidence and recommendations for action', *British Dental Journal*, 187: 6–12.

Weeks K.J., Milson K.M. and Lennon, M.A. (1993) 'Enamel defects in 4-year-old to 5-year-old children in fluoridated and non-fluoridated parts of Cheshire, UK', *Caries Research*, 27: 317–20.

Wilson, K.I. (1992) 'Treatment accessibility for physically and mentally handicapped people – a review of the literature', *Community Dental Health*, 9: 187–92.

Yiamouyiannis, J.A. (1983) *Fluoride: The Aging Factor*. Delware: Health Action Press.

Zimmerman, M., Bornstein, R. and Martinsson, T. (1995) 'Utilization of dental services in refugees in Sweden 1975–1985', *Community Dentistry and Oral Epidemiology*, 23: 95–9.

Chapter 10

Evaluation and access

*Myfanwy Morgan, Martin Gulliford and
Meryl Hudson*

Introduction

Evaluation of access addresses a range of questions, including:
- Are performance targets in relation to access being achieved?
- Is there inequality in the use of services by different population groups, and how do these relate to need? Why do these inequalities exist?
- How can the organisation of services be changed so as to improve timeliness and appropriateness of utilisation especially for under-served groups?
- How has the introduction of a new service altered patterns of utilisation of existing and new services? What have been the consequences for inequalities in utilisation? How acceptable is the new service to users? What are the health outcomes and how are these distributed between different groups?

Evaluation of access to health care therefore involves monitoring health service structure and performance as well as evaluating new policies and innovations in services. A logical sequence of studies might be used to evaluate whether existing services are achieving their objectives, explain why problems exist, and develop and evaluate new policies and service innovations which address problems in access. Evaluations may be implemented at different levels including the macro-level of the population or health system, the meso-level of the health service organisational unit or district, and the micro-level of the individual practitioner or patient. A range of disciplinary approaches may be adopted (Fulop *et al.* 2001). In this chapter we provide a brief overview with examples of these approaches, and we refer readers to methodological texts for further detail. We first consider methods used for monitoring access. The following section discusses recent developments in the evaluation of users' views of services. Finally we discuss different approaches to the evaluation of innovations in services.

Monitoring and auditing access

Monitoring access involves the assessment of relevant aspects of health service structure and performance. This is undertaken for four main purposes:

- achieving the accountability of health systems (for example, monitoring whether health care plans in the US and hospital trusts in the NHS are providing appropriate access to health care in terms of the availability of services and rates of use);
- monitoring whether specific policy targets have been met (for example, targets for waiting times for services, uptake of preventive care, population insurance coverage);
- monitoring whether the health service is achieving the goal of equity in relation to the availability and use of services by socio-economic, ethnic, gender and other social groupings;
- assessing consumer acceptability and satisfaction with the access to services as part of a wider consumer evaluation of services.

Monitoring access is of interest to policy-makers, planners and managers and the general public. It forms part of a policy process and it is also a basis for research to examine the reasons for apparent variations in uptake or divergence from targets.

Data sources

The Institute of Medicine's report, *Access to Health Care in America*, provides a detailed review of the development of indicators of access (Millman 1993).

Appropriate data may be obtained through routine information collected for administrative or monitoring purposes. These include data on hospital referrals, uptake of preventive services, inpatient admissions and waiting times. Other data are collected through regular and special surveys of the general population or specific client groups, and by eliciting users' or the general public's views of access through established feedback mechanisms. Routinely collected data generally include few health status measures which can be used to evaluate the outcomes of care. Mortality data provide valuable insights and are especially useful in the evaluation of some clinical areas such as cancer treatment services (Quinn *et al.* 1988). Other clinical outcome measures are generally poorly recorded in routine data and this has led to the development of a number of specialised clinical databases in specialist areas such as cardiac surgery or intensive care (Black 1997). Subjective measures of health status, including generic measures like the Short Form 36 questionnaire and condition-specific scales, are increasingly incorporated into patient and population surveys. However, results obtained using these measures are not easily translated into policy-relevant formats (Patrick and Erickson 1993).

Routinely collected data, and data from surveys, are used to obtain information about the availability, utilisation and outcomes of services. These data may be analysed at a national level but the population may also be segmented into groups according to geographical or administrative units, insurance status, ethnicity, or socio-economic status. Other analyses may be by condition or client groups (examples include coronary heart disease, cancer, or children), or in relation to type of health care organisation and funding (health authority, hospital or primary care trust in the UK, or type of funder or service provider in a mixed economy of care).

Methods of analysis

At the simplest level, rates of access may be compared for different population groups using absolute measures, such as differences in rates, or relative measures based on rate ratios. Such routine indicators provide fairly crude data that can give information on trends and alert managers and policy-makers to possible problems in the performance of health systems. Difficulties of interpretation may arise from concerns about the quality of the original data or the occurrence in some cases of only small numbers of events. The ranking of indicators in the form of league tables is considered to provide incentives to performance but may be misleading because the estimates are themselves imprecise, and confidence intervals will often show substantial overlap in the results for different units (Goldstein and Speigelhalter 1996). Regression methods offer a flexible approach that permits estimation of measures of access after adjustment for measures of need or case mix. Measures of need will usually include relevant health status measures, and adjustment for need will usually be performed to evaluate inequities in the utilisation of care (see Chapter 3). Case-mix measures typically include information about important prognostic variables including demographic and social characteristics, the presence of associated diseases or co-morbidities, and measures of the severity of illness. Case-mix adjustment will usually be used to evaluate inequities in the outcomes of care. More sophisticated analyses require a multi-level framework to allow for the correlation of responses within areas or organisational units (Goldstein and Speigelhalter 1996). Measures based on the concentration index may be estimated as summary measures of inequality and inequity (Mackenbach and Kunst 1997). Finally, the extent of inequalities may also be contrasted with measures of the impact of inequalities on the population overall. Thus the estimation of measures related to the population attributable risk takes into account not just the magnitude of the inequalities, but also the size of the affected groups (see Chapter 3 for further discussion).

Accountability and performance targets

Emphasis is now given to performance monitoring as a means of improving the quality and efficiency of care. This has been associated in the UK with the recording and publishing of the ratings of hospitals, primary care organisations and health authorities on a range of indicators and rewarding those with above average performance. There are a number of sources of targets and performance indicators, including the NHS performance assessment framework which includes 'Fair access' as one of six dimensions of performance (NHS Executive 2001). Specific targets and indicators for each dimension of performance are specified and employed at national and local level as bench marks to monitor performance. Those relating to fair access currently include ensuring that 60 per cent of patients wait no more than 24 hours for an appointment with a primary health care professional and no more than 48 hours for an appointment with a general practitioner by March 2002; making sure that everyone will be able to see an NHS dentist by phoning NHS Direct by September 2001; and implementing a maximum waiting time for inpatient admission of 15 months by March 2002 and a maximum waiting time of 26 weeks for outpatients (see Chapter 5, Figure 5.1). Other performance indicators include those concerned to monitor the effective delivery of appropriate care and health outcomes. They include the level of potentially 'avoidable hospitalisations' as a result of conditions which should at least in part be treatable in primary care and the level of detection and appropriate prescribing for mental health conditions in primary care, and 'avoidable mortality' indicators such as breast and cervical survival and deaths in hospital following a heart attack, fractured hip or surgery (Department of Health 2001a). National service frameworks are also being developed in the NHS as one of a number of measures to raise quality and decrease variations in services. These involve setting standards of care for a defined service or care group and establishing performance milestones against which a programme within an agreed timescale will be measured.

Specific indicators of performance employed in other health systems also reflect particular policy and programme goals and concerns. For example, budget cuts in Canada have led to considerable emphasis on monitoring the effects of reforms on access to care both for the population as a whole and for vulnerable groups such as people with low socio-economic status and older people (Brownell *et al.* 2001). In the US particular emphasis has been given to performance review and the publication of indicators of quality to ensure that the services provided under various schemes, including to Medicare and Medicaid beneficiaries, meet certain minimum standards of quality, and to selecting and rewarding best performers (Gold 1998; Bodenheimer 1999). Performance indicators also enable purchasers and consumers of health care to choose between plans (National Committee for Quality Assurance 2002).

Programme monitoring involves the use of multiple indicators that may relate to the three domains of access to care, treatment process and outcomes. Utilisation rates generally form the main indicator of access, but may be complemented by indicators of consumer satisfaction, geographical location of services and the ability to afford services. Programme monitoring in the health field has been important in the US and involves the monitoring of particular services such as mental health (Pandiani *et al.* 2002). There are also health-tracking initiatives to report on changes in the US health care system and assess how these changes affect the population's health care. This involves information collected from a number of sources, including a longitudinal study of selected communities across the country (Ginsburg *et al.* 1995). A similar framework for monitoring the impacts of health reforms especially in terms of their impacts on equity has been proposed for Canada, with specific indicators of access including physician contact, rates of hospital admissions and hospital days per capita, rates of surgical procedures and by type, use of diagnostic services and pharmaceuticals, and patients' and the public's views of access (Brownell *et al.* 2001).

Views of service users

Health systems increasingly attempt to obtain the views of the general public and patients as a means of monitoring health service performance and improving the delivery of health care. This includes providing patient feedback on various aspects of the accessibility and the delivery of health care to complement utilisation data, seeking lay views in determining health service priorities (see Chapter 11), and evaluating innovations in service provision from the perspective of users (see review of patient-based approaches in Wensing and Elwyn 2002).

The commitment in the NHS to incorporating lay views is described in a discussion document, *Involving Patients and the Public in Healthcare* (Department of Health 2001b). This set out proposals for implementing the vision of a patient-centred NHS outlined in the National Plan, with the aim to 'move away from a system of patients being on the outside, to one where the voices of patients, their carers and the public generally are heard and listened to through every level of the service, acting as a lever for change and improvement' (Department of Health 2001b). This section focuses on patients' involvement in monitoring and evaluating services in terms of providing feedback and expressing opinions on service availability, accessibility and quality.

Membership of committees and groups

There are currently proposals within the NHS to create new structures that provide a more powerful system than previously for involving patients and the public in health (Department of Health 2001b). This includes establishing Patient Forums that are intended to be 'truly representative of a broad sweep of the community' in every acute hospital and primary care trust. Patient Forums will be statutory independent bodies made up of patients and others from the local community, with the remit of finding out what patients and carers think about the services they use, monitoring the quality of services from the patient perspective and working with the local NHS trust to bring about improvements. These groups have a wide remit, to include satisfaction with the accessibility of services in relation to the needs of diverse groups in the population, as well as various dimensions of the quality of care. As Coulter (2002) cautions, while most patients want providers to take account of their views and experiences, there is a problem that only a small unrepresentative minority will want to be actively involved in committees to achieve this. It will therefore be crucial to ensure that the Patient Forums have access to regular feedback from representative samples of patients and citizens to balance the views of special interest groups, and ensure that patients'/ citizens' views are adequately taken into account at the stage of service development.

Surveys of public or user views

Surveys involve the collection of information using a fairly structured questionnaire. This generally involves self-completed postal surveys but may involve interviews administered face-to-face or telephone interviews, with telephone surveys being particularly commonly used in the US. Surveys (especially postal) enable the views and experiences of large numbers of people to be collected fairly quickly and cheaply and analysed by age, sex, socio-economic group or region. A limitation is that low response rates may introduce a bias, especially as this tends to be highest among more disadvantaged groups in the population. Achieving relatively high response rates requires consideration of the length of questionnaire, mode of distribution, and translation into appropriate languages (for a review of survey methods see Bowling 2000). High rates of non-response by particular groups may also require that the sample is weighted to derive population estimates (Zaslowsky et al. 2002).

Major national surveys to collect data on patients' views and experience of health care include three independent national studies conducted by the Johnson Foundation in the US in 1976, 1982 and 1986 using telephone interviews. These surveys aimed to measure the extent to which individuals were experiencing problems in obtaining medical care and to examine changes over time (Freeman et al. 2002). More recently there has been an emphasis on identifying the insured population's satisfaction with managed care plans. These now account for more than half of the employed insured population in the US and restrict enrolees' choice of access to a network of physicians, hospitals and other providers (Davis et al. 1995). In England a series of national patient surveys was instituted in 1997 to contribute to monitoring the performance of the NHS as seen from the patient's perspective and to enable systematic comparisons to be made of experiences over time and between different parts of the country. The first survey in this programme was the 1998 General Practice Survey which covered a range of issues including patients' experiences and views regarding access and waiting times, out-of-hours care, and the helpfulness and availability of surgery staff including practice nurses and receptionists. This survey was based on a sample of 1,000 people randomly selected from each of the 100 Health Authorities in England and was completed by 61.4 per cent. Subsequent surveys in this programme have been based on coronary heart disease patients and cancer patients.

In the US health plans are required to survey their members, using a common instrument, about their experiences with their health plan (Edgman-Levitan and

Cleary 1996). Every trust in England is also now required to survey their patients annually as part of an audit/monitoring programme. Patient assessments also frequently form an aspect of the local audit of primary care services in the NHS. A published example from one inner city practice aimed to access patients' satisfaction with primary health care. Self-completed questionnaires were completed for 248 attenders and 74 home interviews were conducted for those who had requested house calls (Hannay et al. 1997). This provided information on satisfaction with care provided by the practice, including referral to hospital for specialist treatment, difficulties in contacting a doctor and visits by the primary care team for patients who were housebound, and the types of services that patients thought should be available in the health centre (including physiotherapist, chiropodist and pharmacist).

A common limitation of surveys to assess patients' views and satisfaction with access and the quality of services is that small differences in question wording, including the extent to which users' perceptions and views are elicited using negative statements, influence responses and thus reduce possibilities for comparison (Cohen et al. 1996). Many instruments employed in earlier studies were also based on researcher-defined views of relevant dimensions. This may not correspond with patients' own concerns and priorities and a greater number of validated patient-centred instruments informed by data derived from focus groups or in-depth interviews are now available. An example is the General Practice Assessment Survey (GPAS) from the National Primary Care Research and Development Centre at the University of Manchester. GPAS is a patient-completed questionnaire that asks about aspects of general practice care, including access and communication, where patient views are an essential part of finding out about quality, and collects both factual data on patients' experiences and subjective ratings of quality. GPAS is now employed by a number of primary care groups and trusts across the UK to assess the quality of care in their practices, and national benchmark data have been developed from these surveys (Ramsay et al. 2000).

Patient-based evaluations raise questions regarding the interpretation of ratings of 'satisfaction'. This appears to be strongly influenced by patient expectations that are in turn derived from their own or other people's prior experiences (normative or comparative expectations) and the care they would like or hope for (idealised expectations) (McKinley et al. 2002). Differences in ratings by different socio-economic, age, sex and cultural groups or between services and types of care may therefore be confounded by a match or mismatch between expectations and access to care or other aspects of quality. In order to overcome this problem, a measure developed by the Picker/Commonwealth Program for Patient Centered Care emphasises the collection of factual data of patients' experiences with a particular provider, rather than more general views and subjective evaluations. For example it asks how long people had waited rather than whether this was too long or not. These patient reports therefore reflect their observations rather than their evaluations but can be used to identify areas that require quality improvement. The Picker inpatient survey has been used in the US, Canada and several European health systems including the NHS. This identifies access (time spent waiting for admission and time between admission and allocation to the ward) as one of eight dimensions of patient-centred care. A similar approach has been used to develop measures for use in primary care, outpatient, accident and emergency and other settings (www.pickereurope.org/surveys).

Evaluation of innovations in services

During the 1990s a predominant policy concern was with increasing the efficiency of health services. In the research field, this led to a preoccupation with evaluations of clinical effectiveness and cost-effectiveness in health care in which the random-ised controlled trial was considered as the optimal design for the evaluation of innovations. Such studies generally provided little evidence for the distributional consequences of different choices in service provision or clinical practice. A recent review suggested that 'existing economic evaluations do not represent an adequate guide to resource allocation decisions when the distributional effects of such decisions may be relevant' (Sassi *et al.* 2001: iv). Sassi *et al.* (2001) suggested that researchers involved in evaluating services should at least collect information about the characteristics of the populations likely to benefit from the service, and the likely effectiveness and cost-effectiveness of the service for different groups in the population. A related problem has been that most effort has been devoted to defining what is the 'right service', rather than to evaluating how the service should be organised and delivered so as to achieve optimal utilisation and outcomes (Sheldon 2001). This section briefly considers the application of randomised designs in the evaluation of access to care; we then discuss alternative models of evaluation that are particularly suited to examining the impacts of organisational changes.

Randomised controlled trials

Randomised controlled trials involve data collected before and after the intervention and are therefore longitudinal in nature. A key characteristic is the random allocation of units to the intervention or control groups. Randomisation may be at the level of the individual subject or at the level of the geographical area or health service organisational unit. Studies in which the unit of allocation is a cluster of individuals are increasingly applied but are often statistically inefficient and require special considerations in design and analysis (Donner and Klar 2000; Ukoumunne *et al.* 1999). Innovations to improve access will usually be 'complex' in the sense that they include several components. Such interventions are difficult to evaluate because they are hard to define, develop and reproduce. A group convened by the UK Medical Research Council suggested that a phased approach to evaluation should be adopted. An initial phase requiring the integration of theory, modelling and observational data is used to develop and define the intervention, leading on to an exploratory trial, before a definitive trial is undertaken (Campbell *et al.* 2000).

In many randomised controlled trials of new health service interventions, access is not included as a relevant outcome. For example, a recent systematic review of evaluations of nurse practitioners in primary care found that studies included in the review reported measures of patient satisfaction, quality of care, and health status but not measures of access (Horrocks *et al.* 2002). However, some randomised controlled trials have used access to health care, and patients' use of services, as the chosen measures of effect. One group of studies focused on the evaluation of information provision to patients with the aim of improving the uptake of preventive medical services such as breast screening (Richards *et al.* 2001). Other studies tried to modify patients' help-seeking behaviours. Little *et al.* (2001) reported a trial which evaluated the use of an information booklet to increase the appropriateness of patients' use of primary care services for minor illnesses. Randomised trials have also addressed financial barriers to access. Perhaps the best known example is the Rand Health Insurance Experiment already referred to in Chapters 6 and 8. In this study, families were randomly allocated to different forms of health insurance that either provided free health care, or required some cost-sharing in which patients contributed towards the cost of care. The study showed that utilisation of physician visits and hospital inpatient services were lower in the cost-sharing group, but overall health outcomes were similar in the two groups (Brook *et al.* 1983; Newhouse *et al.* 1981).

Randomised studies addressing organisational barriers to access have mostly been conducted at the level of the practice or practitioner. An example is a study in which general practitioners were provided with a risk factor checklist and a training video in order to improve the appropriateness of their referral of children with suspected otitis media with effusion. Here there may be a barrier to appropriate access of specialist services, both because general practitioners may fail to refer children who need specialist attention, and because inappropriate referrals may increase waiting times for those who need attention. The authors found that these educational interventions increased the appropriateness of GPs' referrals to secondary care (Bennett *et al.* 2001). The requirement for replication will often present prohibitive logistical or resource requirements for randomised studies at higher or more complex organisational levels. However, Black (2001) concluded that decision-making processes in relation to policies on service organisation and delivery seldom sought or used rigorous research evidence. For example, randomised evaluations were not sought for general practitioner fundholding schemes in the UK.

Alternative approaches to evaluation

Changes in health policy, or in methods for organising and delivering services, often have important implications for access but such interventions are not often the subject of randomised evaluations. When randomised trials are carried out they may not provide a suitable setting for the evaluation of access issues because the conduct of a trial may require that access be constrained, either through the selection of subjects or through the delivery of the intervention. Non-randomised studies therefore play a major role in the evaluation of access. Among non-randomised studies a distinction can be made between those in which the allocation of the intervention was made by the investigator, and those in which the investigators were passive observers of the consequences of changes in policy at local, regional or national level. The former might be termed quasi-experimental, while the latter would more often be regarded as observational studies. Further discussion of design issues is provided by Cook and Campbell (1979).

An example of a comparative observational study is an evaluation of a national telephone helpline. This was introduced in England in 1997, with the apparent aims of improving the provision of information to people caring for either their own or their families' illnesses, and limiting the demand on other emergency services. Did provision of access to a telephone helpline result in changes in the utilisation of other emergency services? Munro *et al.* (2000) undertook a comparative observational study based on three geographical areas receiving the newly introduced helpline, and six nearby general practitioner cooperatives as controls. General practitioner cooperatives represent groupings of general practices that share responsibility for providing out-of-hours services. On comparing trends in the use of emergency services before and after the introduction of the helpline, the authors found that there were no changes in the utilisation of accident and emergency departments or ambulance services, but there was a small deceleration in the trend towards increased use of general practitioner out-of-hours services. This helpline has now been rolled out as a national service and followed by descriptive evaluations of the operation of the service in terms of patterns of use, patient-reported barriers to care, acceptability and satisfaction, the appropriateness of advice and demands on other services.

Models of evaluation deriving from other disciplinary approaches are considered in detail by Fulop and colleagues (2001) and include economic evaluation, operational research, policy analysis, action research and qualitative studies. These approaches, rather than evaluating a controlled experiment, build models which can then be tested (operational research and organisational psychology and also applicable to economics) or use everyday or natural sources of data as their contexts (organisational studies, sociology and policy analysis). Each approach can address different questions arising from a change in service delivery.

Resource constraints and the concern to increase hospital activity, and thus patient access to services, have increased the importance of modelling approaches in examining the impacts of changes in service delivery. This is exemplified by research to model the effects of booked inpatient admissions on capacity requirements for an intensive care unit. The results suggested that such systems may result in frequent operational difficulties if there is a high degree of variability in length of stay and reserve capacity is limited. Both of these limitations exist in the NHS (Gallivan *et al.* 2002).

The introduction of complex service innovations to increase access and improve the quality of care often involves a package of changes in service delivery that may have multiple objectives and affect more than one level in the system. Examples include integrated diabetes care schemes, rapid access clinics and community outreach services, and national service frameworks for particular diseases and care groups. It is increasingly recognised that the effects of such innovations depend on the specific context, including aspects of the community or organisational setting, such as patient characteristics, staff levels and turnover, staff views and commitment to the innovation and channels of communication and so on. While these local factors may compromise the generalisability of an innovation, collection of relevant data may contribute to an understanding of the ways in which they contribute to its success or failure. Evaluation therefore requires to be broadly based to acquire an understanding of mechanisms, context and outcomes, in terms of why a programme or model of service provision works, for whom, and in what circumstances, in order to refine future innovations and initiatives. This accords with Pawson and Tilley's (1997) notion of 'realistic evaluation' and Weiss and colleagues' theory of change approach in relation to community-based initiatives (Connell et al. 1995). These approaches are not yet well developed in the health field, but are beginning to inform the evaluation of community-based programmes, such as the evaluation of Health Action Zones that have been set up in disadvantaged areas in the UK to address health inequalities (Judge 2000). More generally, evaluations of complex service interventions are typically characterised by the use of qualitative methods of data collection (semi-structured/in-depth interviews, focus groups or participant observation) to complement quantitative data on inputs and outcomes, and examine processes and procedures and the perspectives and experiences of key stakeholders (Murphy and Dingwall 1998; Barbour 1999). One approach that is receiving increased attention in the health field is action research, which has been widely used to facilitate change in industry (Bate 2000). This approach combines quantitative and qualitative methods with the aim of making improvements by working with staff in the organisation in a cycle of action, data gathering, analysis, reflection, and planning further action. The aim is to establish not merely if something works but how it works and how things can be improved, and has been described as involving a shift from evaluation for judgement to evaluation for learning (Carter et al. 1995).

Conclusions

This chapter outlines a variety of methods and approaches that are now employed in monitoring access to care, and in developing and evaluating new innovations and initiatives to promote access at either primary care or hospital level. Important changes have included a greater emphasis on eliciting patient and provider views, and concerns with process as well as outcomes. However, despite an increase in activity, many locally-based initiatives designed to increase the accessibility and quality of care have not been formally evaluated (Atkinson et al. 2001). There is also a need to synthesise the evidence derived from different approaches to the evaluation of particular innovations and initiatives, with each approach contributing in different ways to an understanding of complex service developments.

References

Barbour, R. (1999) 'The case for combining qualitative and quantitative approaches in health services research', *Journal of Health Services Research and Policy*, 4: 39–43.

Bate, P. (2000) Synthesizing research and practice: using the action research approach in health care settings. *Social Policy and Administration*, 34(4): 478–93.

Bennett. K., Haggard, M., Churchill, R. and Wood, S. (2001) 'Improving referrals for glue ear from primary care: are multiple interventions better than one alone?', *Journal of Health Services Research and Policy*, 6: 139–44.

Black, N.A. (1997) 'Developing high-quality clinical databases. The key to a new research paradigm', *British Medical Journal*, 315: 831–2.

Black, N. (2001) 'Evidence-based policy: proceed with care', *British Medical Journal*, 323: 275–9.

Bodenheimer, T. (1999) 'The movement for improved quality in health care', *The New England Journal of Medicine*, 340: 488–92.

Bowling, A. (2000) *Research Methods in Health*. Buckingham: Open University Press.

Brook, R.H., Ware, J.E., Rogers, W.H., Keeler, E.B., Davies, A.R., Donald, C.A., Goldberg, G.A., Lohr, K.N., Masthay, P.C. and Newhouse, J.P. (1983) 'Does free care improve adult health – results from a randomized controlled trial', *New England Journal of Medicine*, 309(23): 1426–34.

Brownell, M.D., Roos, N.P. and Roos, L.L. (2001) 'Monitoring health reform: a report card approach', *Social Science and Medicine*, 52: 657–70.

Campbell, M., Fitzpatrick, R., Haines, A., Kinmonth, A.L., Sandercock, P., Spiegelhalter, D.J. and Tyrer, P. (2000) 'Framework for design and evaluation of complex interventions to improve health', *British Medical Journal*, 321: 694–6.

Carter, N., Klein, R. and Day, P. (1995) *How Organizations Measure Success: The Use of Performance Indicators in Government*. London: Routledge.

Cohen, G., Forbes, J. and Garraway, M. (1996) 'Can different patient satisfaction survey methods yield consistent results? Comparison of three surveys', *British Medical Journal*, 313: 841–4.

Connell, J.P., Kubisch, A.C., Schorr, L.B and Weiss, C.H. (1995) *New Approaches to Evaluating Community Initiatives: Concepts, Methods and Contexts*. Washington, DC: The Aspen Institute.

Cook, T.D. and Campbell, D.T. (1979), *Quasi-experimentation. Design and analysis issues for field settings*. Chicago: Rand McNally College Publishing Company.

Coulter, A. (ed.) (2002) 'Involving patients: representation or representativeness?', *Health Expectations*, 5: 1.

Davis, K., Scott Collins, K., Schoen, C. and Morris, C. (1995) 'Choice matters: enrollees' views of their health plans', *Health Affairs*, 14: 99–112.

Department of Health (2001a) *Quality and Performance in the NHS: High Level Performance and Clinical Indicators* London: Department of Health. http://www.doh. gov.uk/indicat/indicat.htm; accessed September 24 2001.

Department of Health (2001b) *Involving Patients and the Public in Healthcare: Response to the Listening Exercise*. London: Department of Health.

Donner, A. and Klar, N. (2000) *Design and Analysis of Cluster Randomisation Trials*. London: Arnold.

Edgman-Levitan, S. and Cleary, P.D. (1996) 'What information do consumers want?', *Health Affairs*, 15: 42–56.

Freeman, H.E., Blendon, R.J., Aiken, L.H., Sudman, S., Connie, F.M and Corey, C.R. (2002) 'Americans report on their access to health care', *Health Affairs*, 21: 6–18.

Fulop, N., Allen, P., Clarke, A. and Black, N. (2001) *Studying the Organisation and Delivery of Health Services: Research Methods*. London: Routledge.

Gallivan, S., Utley, M., Treasure, T. and Valencia, O. (2002) 'Booked inpatient admissions and hospital capacity: mathematical modelling study', *British Medical Journal*, 324: 280–2.

Ginsburg, B., Hughes, R.G. and Knickman, J.R. (1995) 'Special report: a Robert Wood Johnson program to monitor health system change', *Health Affairs*, 14: 287–91.

Gold, M. (1998) 'The concept of access and managed care', *Health Services Research*, 33: 625–52.

Goldstein, H. and Spiegelhalter, D.J. (1996) 'League tables and their limitations: statistical issues in comparisons of institutional performance', *Journal of the Royal Statistical Society, A*, 159: 385–443.

Hannay, D.R., Sunners, C.M. and Platts, M. (1997) 'Patient perceptions of primary care in an inner-city practice', *Family Practice*, 14: 355–60.

Horrocks, S., Anderson, E. and Salisbury, C. (2002) 'Systematic review of whether nurse practitioners working in primary care can provide equivalent care to doctors', *British Medical Journal*, 324: 819–23.

Judge, K. (2000) 'Testing evaluation to the limits', *Journal of Health Services Research and Policy*, 5(1): 3–5.

Little, P., Somerville, J., Williamson, I., Warner, G., Moore, M., Wiles, R., George, S., Smith, A. and Peveler, R. (2001) 'Randomised controlled trial of self management leaflets and booklets for minor illness provided by post', *British Medical Journal*, 322(7296): 1214–17.

Mackenbach, J.P. and Kunst, A.E. (1997) 'Measuring the magnitude of socio-economic inequalities in health: an overview of available measures illustrated with two examples from Europe', *Social Science and Medicine*, 44: 757–71.

McKinley, R., Stevenson, K., Adams, S. and Manku-Scott, T. (2002) 'Meeting patient expectations of care: the major determinant of satisfaction with out-of-hours primary medical care?', *Family Practice*, 19: 333–8.

Millman, M. (1993) *Access to Health Care in America*. Washington, DC: National Academy Press.

Munro, J., Nicholl, J., O'Cathain, A. and Knowles, E. (2000) 'Impact of NHS Direct on demand for immediate care: observational study', *British Medical Journal*, 321(7254): 150–3.

Murphy, E. and Dingwall, R. (1998) 'Qualitative methods in health services research'. In N. Black, J. Brazier, R. Fitzpatrick, B. Reeves (eds) *Health Services Research Methods: A Guide to Best Practice*. London: BMJ Books.

National Committee for Quality Assurance (2002) *Health Plan Employer Data and Information Set*. Washington, DC: National Committee for Quality Assurance. Available at http://www.ncqa.org/communications/publications/hedispub.htm; accessed 16 August 2002.

National Health Service Executive (2001) *The New NHS Modern and Dependable: A National Framework for Assessing Performance*. Consultation Document. Leeds: NHS Executive.

Newhouse, J.P., Manning, W.G., Morris, C.N., Orr, L.L., Duan, N., Keeler, E.B., Leibowitz, A., Marquis, K.H., Marquis, M.S., Phelps, C.E. and Brook, R.H. (1981) 'Some interim results from a controlled trial of cost-sharing in health-insurance', *New England Journal of Medicine*, 305: 1501–7.

Pandiani, J.A., Banks, S.M., Bramley, J., Pomeroy, S. and Simon, M. (2002) 'Measuring access to mental health care: a multi-indicator approach to program evaluation', *Evaluation and Program Planning* 25: 271-85

Patrick, D. and Erickson, P. (1993) *Health Status and Health Policy. Quality of Life in Health Care Evaluation and Resource Allocation*. Oxford: Oxford University Press.

Pawson, R. and Tilley, N. (1997) *Realistic Evaluation*. London: Sage.

Quinn, M.J., Martinez-Garcia, C. and Berrino, F. (1988) 'Variations in survival from breast cancer in Europe by age and country', 1978–1989', *European Journal of Cancer*, 34: 2204–11.

Ramsay, J., Campbell, J.L., Schroter, J., Green, J. and Roland, R. (2000) 'The general practice assessment survey (GPAS): tests of data quality and measurement properties', *Family Practice*, 17: 372–9.

Richards, S.H., Bankhead, C., Peters, T.J., Austoker, J., Hobbs, F.D.R., Brown, J., Tydeman, C., Roberts, L., Formby, J., Redman, V., Wilson, S. and Sharp, D.J. (2001) 'Cluster randomised controlled trial comparing the effectiveness and cost-effectiveness of two primary care interventions aimed at improving attendance for breast screening', *Journal of Medical Screening*, 8: 91–8.

Sassi, F., Archard, L. and Le Grand, J. (2001) 'Equity and the economic evaluation of health care', *Health Technology Assessment*, 5: 3.

Sheldon, T.A. (2001) 'It ain't what you do but the way that you do it', *Journal of Health Services Research Policy*, 6: 3–5.

Ukoumunne, O.C., Gulliford, M.C., Chinn, S., Sterne, J.A.C. and Burney, P.G.J. (1999) 'Methods for evaluating area-wide and organisation-based interventions in health and health care. A methodological systematic review for the NHS Research and Development Health Technology Assessment Programme', *Health Technology Assessment*, 3: 5.

Wensing, M. and Elwyn, G. (2002) 'Research on patients' views in the evaluation and improvement of quality in care', *Quality and Safety in Health Care*, 11: 153–7.

Zaslowsky, A.M., Zaborshi, L.B. and Cleary, P.D. (2002) 'Factors affecting response rates to consumer assessment of health plans study', *Medical Care*, 40: 485–99.

Chapter 11

Reform, rationing and choice in a changing context

Martin Gulliford and Myfanwy Morgan

The changing context

The goals of improving access to care and achieving equity are set in a rapidly changing medical and social context. Innovations in health technology over the past 30 years include major advances in surgery such as successful hip and knee replacements; the introduction of coronary by-pass surgery, and kidney, heart, lung and other transplant operations; new investigative procedures; and high-cost drug treatments such as antiretroviral therapies for AIDS. The overall effect of new possibilities for treatment is an expansion of medical needs and the potential for health care. Needs for services are further increased by the advancing age of the population and the success of medicine in extending the lives of patients with chronic conditions. A larger proportion of the population now experiences chronic or degenerative conditions that will benefit from treatment to improve functioning, reduce pain and enhance the quality of life. Costly procedures that were initially evaluated on younger patients often diffuse into health care for the elderly, thus further increasing demands for services (Dozet *et al.* 2002). The scope of preventive activities has also expanded through developments in antenatal and newborn screening, child health checks and immunisations, cancer screening techniques and new preventive measures such as cholesterol screening and regular health checks for elderly people.

There have also been important social changes. On the one hand, a majority of people have increasing knowledge and expectations of health care and want to participate in health decisions. At the same time there are growing sectors of the population which experience relative disadvantage and social exclusion associated with poverty, unemployment, long-term illness, recent migration status and other social circumstances. These groups have the greatest needs for health care but often experience the greatest problems gaining access to services. Thus while the overall level of access has increased, there has also been an increase in the potential for inequality and inequity. This is illustrated by the increase in socioeconomic inequality in mortality from coronary heart disease which occurred while overall mortality rates from this condition declined and opportunities for primary and secondary prevention increased (Kawachi *et al.* 1991).

Advances in medical technologies, the changing health needs of the population and increasing public and patient expectations together with price inflation in health services have had the effect of increasing health care costs. Health care expenditure as a proportion of national income has progressively increased over time, reaching nearly 13 per cent of gross domestic product (GDP) in the USA in 1998. In the UK, the Wanless report suggested that health spending needed to increase from 7.7 per cent of GDP in 2002 to reach a figure of 11.1 per cent, closer to the European average, in 2022 (Wanless 2002).

Health care reform

A general response to the need to reconcile supply and demand for services has been to shift to a more efficiency-driven perspective in which the market mechanism has increasingly taken priority over the equity focus of previous generations. This emphasis on cost-effectiveness and efficiency has been justified as a necessary response to increasing cost pressures. The desire to increase efficiency was not the only motivation for reforms of health services implemented in many countries during the 1990s, others included improving responsiveness to consumers and increasing choice, but these reforms typically included packages of measures designed to regulate, or introduce competition into, the production and consumption of health care (Saltman *et al.* 1998). The separation of purchasing and provider functions, development of markets for services, increased use of cost-sharing measures, promotion of clinical effectiveness and quality assurance, and elimination of ineffective and low-priority treatments all aimed to increase the efficiency of service utilisation. An illustration is provided in the various strategies implemented to control the growth of expenditures on pharmaceuticals which now account for between 10 per cent and 20 per cent of health expenditures in European countries (Mossialos 1998). On the demand side, some measures were directed at patients. These included increased cost-sharing, increased licensing of products for over the counter sale, and also public education measures to reduce the consumption of drugs. Other interventions were directed at pharmacists and physicians including financial measures such as changes to payment mechanisms and allocation of fixed budgets for prescribing, and clinical measures to increase the appropriateness of prescribing through the use of clinical guidelines and audits of prescribing patterns. Regulation on the supply side included the implementation of price controls and the introduction of either positive or negative lists of drugs that might, or might not, be prescribed.

These measures illustrate how health policy-makers attempted to contain costs by retreating from the notion of a fully comprehensive service, and by diluting the notion of solidarity through increased individual responsibility for health care. Excluding low-priority treatments of doubtful effectiveness, or care for seemingly low-priority groups such as old mentally impaired people, from the package of services offered through the publicly funded system set a limit on either the comprehensiveness or the universality of the system. Increased cost-sharing gave greater responsibility to individuals for the consumption of pharmaceuticals or dental care (Chapter 8). The exclusion of procedures like in vitro fertilisation from publicly funded care is on the grounds that these should always be the responsibility of the individuals (Klein *et al.* 1995). Rather than a universal, comprehensive system, 'an adequate level of care without excessive burdens' (President's Commission 1983: page 4) appears to be the unstated but more pragmatic objective for most health systems, although there are wide variations in the way this is interpreted.

The requirement for rationing

A concern about lack of access, and inequity in access, requires increased resources for health care, but a desire to control costs leads to the introduction of measures which restrict access to some types of care, or require increased personal financial contributions for others. Vertical equity of access may be compromised because patients with some types of problem will be denied access. Horizontal equity may also be compromised because people with similar needs may not be similarly able to gain access to services. In a geographical context this is exemplified by the tension between the wish to centralise services in order to provide economies of scale, as compared with the desire to protect access for those who are distant from the central service. In a therapeutic context, this is exemplified by the conflict between the desire to increase the use of effective but costly new drugs like statins through national standards for prescribing, while at the same time requiring control of total prescribing costs. In the context of elective services, there is a desire to limit waiting times to the minimum, while safeguarding the appropriateness of service utilisation and avoiding the inefficiency of surplus capacity.

A fundamental problem in the provision of publicly funded health services, is that resources are limited but demands are potentially infinite (Maxwell 1995). For politicians, this is reflected in the dilemma of meeting public expectations for improved health services while at the same time prudently restraining public expenditure and the need for taxation. For health policy-makers this raises questions concerning how limited resources can best be used to facilitate access to health care. These considerations focus on rationing as a means of determining which services should be available and who should have access to health care. Maxwell (1995) observed that 'Within the NHS services have been rationed primarily by limiting access in a variety of ways. Waiting lists for elective conditions are the most visible and obvious of these' (page 765).

Rationing has been defined in different ways. In the most general sense, rationing represents the method used to allocate resources when the distribution is not decided by price (Parker 1975). Klein *et al.* (1996) suggested that rationing 'takes place in circumstances when supply is restrained by considerations of cost but demand is not restrained by considerations of price' (page 9). According to these definitions, it is not possible to suggest that rationing might be avoided if additional resources were made available, or if inefficiencies were eradicated (Ham and Honigsbaum 1998). There are two types of rationing: financial rationing in which resources are allocated between different services or different administrative areas, and service rationing in which service providers decide who should receive their services. Klein *et al.* (1996) refer to financial rationing as 'priority setting'.

Priority setting

Concerns about rationing include both the level of resources allocated to health care and the distribution of these resources between different services and population groups. Recent commitments to increase investment in health care in the UK, show that there is a consensus that health services were too severely rationed overall leading to excessive waiting times and a concern that health outcomes might be compromised (Chapters 5 and 6). These ideas are reflected in the priorities set for the NHS through the Department of Health Public Service Agreement which includes three objectives (Downing Street Newsroom 2002). Under the first objective, targets are set for maximum waits of three months for outpatient appointments and six months for inpatient treatments to be achieved by 2005. The second objective concerns targets for improvements in health outcomes in terms of reducing mortality from heart disease and cancer; improving health for the mentally ill, elderly people and children; and improving participation in drug treatment programmes. The third objective concerns value for money and sets a target of a 1 per cent annual improvement in cost efficiency and service effectiveness.

These objectives for access seem to depart from the view that health care should be allocated according to need. Instead limits are set on waiting times that are informed not only by medical considerations but also by what is considered socially or politically acceptable across a range of health problems. A further difficulty with explicit objectives of this nature is that everything that is excluded will receive lower priority. This raises concern for equity between conditions and care groups because some health problems are given priority over others. Furthermore, inequalities in access may not be reduced through the implementation of national targets. Inequalities between local areas may increase if intervention strategies are more effective in areas where health care is already more accessible (Lindholm *et al.* 1996). National strategies need to be complemented by local strategies to reduce inequalities in health and access to care by addressing local priorities. This is recognised in the UK through the requirement for local health bodies to produce 'health improvement programmes'.

In the NHS, allocations to regional and local levels have increasingly been guided by explicit formulae; however, priority-setting decisions made at these levels tend to be strongly influenced by historical configurations of services. Furthermore in the UK, local health authorities are held accountable for national priorities, but are not democratically accountable at the local level. These factors tend to reduce the effectiveness of these bodies at setting local priorities, leading to only marginal changes in the organisation of services. At the level of service delivery, rationing is mainly carried out at the discretion of providers. Waiting lists, clinical guidelines and other eligibility rules may be used to ration health care in a formal way. Long delays and waits, short consultation times and unsympathetic, or even hostile, communication may be used as informal mechanisms to discourage the use of services and restrict the amount of service consumed (Parker 1975).

Methods for priority setting and rationing

Priority setting and rationing decisions are central to the question of access, because they have a direct influence on the availability of services, and the criteria governing how they should be used. In theory, rationing decisions need to be informed in several different ways (see also Chapter 6). Information is needed about the ability of different groups to benefit from health care and about the effectiveness, costs and distributional consequences of different types of health care intervention. This information is provided through the processes of health technology assessment whose results can inform the development of evidence-based guidelines. These results have to be set in the context of the ethical and moral values on which decision-making processes should be made. For example, is it better to maximise 'health gain' for the population by investing in effective treatments, or to protect the rights of all individuals equally by providing needed services which contribute less to overall welfare? The interests of different stakeholder groups, including professionals, managers, politicians, patients and the public, will also inform the decision-making process. In practice, the basis of most rationing decisions has usually remained implicit in the sense that 'resource constraints may often have shaped the decisions of doctors, but the decisions themselves were usually presented to patients as reflecting clinical judgements about their chances of benefiting from treatment' (Klein et al. 1995: 769–70).

In response to public and consumer concerns, rationing decisions are increasingly made in ways that are more explicit, but the best way forward remains uncertain and disputed. Using one approach, decisions are made by groups consisting largely of experts who consider technical and ethical issues and use these either to make decisions, or to decide on the principles on which decisions should be made. This approach is exemplified by the National Institute for Clinical Excellence in the UK which uses technical information to decide whether new treatments should be adopted for use in the NHS. In the Netherlands, the Dutch Government Committee on Choices in Health Care (an de Ven 1995) outlined four criteria that might be used to select the basic package of care to be offered through the mandatory health insurance system. The criteria were that the care must be necessary to meet basic needs, must be effective, must be efficient in the sense that the marginal costs must not be too high if the marginal benefit is small, and must not be a form of care that could be left to individual responsibility.

Public and consumer involvement

Another approach is to engage the public more directly in health care decisions. Public involvement in priority setting is formally endorsed in the UK (National Health Service 1992; Department of Health 1999) and in a number of other countries including Sweden (Swedish Parliamentary Priorities Commission 1995), Finland (Working Group on Health Care Prioritisation 1995) and New Zealand (National Advisory Committee on Core Health and Disability Support Services 1998). This incorporation of public and consumer voices acknowledges the existence of differing values among groups in the population and the importance of involving all stakeholders to enhance the acceptability of priorities and rationing decisions. Public participation is also regarded as promoting democracy and a sense of responsibility among citizens, and of increasing local accountability of medical professionals and managers. However, in practice the form and degree of public influence is variable and undefined. It ranges from citizens being consulted without obligation to act or take notice of their views, to public representatives participating fully within the wider decision-making process. A study in the UK of public attitudes to involvement at different levels of health care decision-making showed there was a strong desire for consultation at both the health system level (determining location of services within the authority) and at the programme level (determining the funding of particular types of specialist services), with the guarantee that their contribution would be heard and that decisions taken following consultation would be explained (Litva *et al.* 2002).

A wide range of methods is now used to obtain the public's views and priorities to inform the development of services and priorities for services. This includes 'mass' approaches such as public meetings and questionnaires. Increasing use is also made of focus groups and rapid appraisal methods to determine community views by interviewing 'key' people deemed to be in touch with local opinion. There are also methods to elicit views from informed citizens through, for example, Citizens' Juries where a 'representative panel' of citizens meets over several days to hear evidence of a particular issue and 'deliver their verdict'. A variety of methodologies are also available for eliciting values and preferences, either explicitly or implicitly, including time trade-off techniques and scaling (see Chapter 6 and Mullen 1999). However, despite important technical developments there remain basic questions about the most appropriate way of recruiting members of the public and the representativeness of those involved, especially of more disadvantaged members of local communities.

There is no country where there is complete satisfaction with access to health care because organising and delivering services will always involve some trade-offs and priority-setting to respond to increasing demands and costs of care. At any one point new issues will arise to challenge prevailing assumptions and structures. This focuses attention on how, and by whom, choices to restrict or facilitate access to health care are made. In the US setting, where these decisions are often made by private insurance companies, Daniels (2000) suggested that decisions should be publicly accessible, based on reasonable principles, subject to appeal when required, and externally regulated. In the setting of predominant public provision of health care, Klein has argued that the important thing is to establish appropriate institutions for making decisions (Klein and Williams 2000). Information on the benefits and costs of health technologies is required, but this will be overshadowed by the values and interests of different stakeholders. Establishing appropriate settings for debate and decision-making should aim to ensure that one particular interest group does not prevail and justice is seen to be done.

Consumer choice and changing policies

The increasing emphasis given to public and consumer involvement in rationing decisions forms one aspect of a more general extension of consumer choice. This also involves increasing participation of lay people in the assessment and evaluation of health services (Chapter 10) and shared decision-making between doctor and patient in individual treatment decisions (Guadagnoli and Ward 1998). There are increasing public expectations of services, and demands from service users for higher standards of care. People are better educated and informed and expect to be treated as consumers rather than patients when using publicly funded services. This emphasises a rational-choice perspective to public policy rather than a collective welfarist perspective (Lindbladh et al. 1998). An example of increasing choice regarding initial health care contacts is discussed by Beech (Chapter 5) in terms of the development of increasingly varied sources of primary care provision in the UK (for example, walk-in clinics, nurse-run telephone help-lines, community pharmacist advisors, etc.) with uptake based on individual choice and local variations in provision.

Current approaches to access in health care depart from the centralised, paternalistic, top-down model which is considered to be characteristic of the welfare state but which is increasingly regarded as both inefficient and unresponsive to consumers. More generally the societal consensus appears to have shifted so that individual autonomy is now ranked more highly than collective responsibility (Lindbladh et al. 1998). At one extreme, Margaret Thatcher famously remarked 'there is no such thing as Society. There are individual men and women, and there are families' (Thatcher 1987). This approach emphasises individual responsibility and meeting individual needs through increased choice in services that are responsive to personal and local situations, circumstances and priorities. This favours the expansion of individual responsibility through private financing and provision of health care. This approach embodies broadly 'libertarian' views, with equity judged through the availability of opportunities and choices rather than the extent to which health care is in practice distributed according to need (Gilson 1998). The concern is that such a course will leave publicly funded health care services to develop as 'poor services for poor people'.

A different approach supports the role of collective responsibility through public financing of health care but acknowledges the possibility of both public and private provision of services organised at the local level. This requires that modernised publicly funded health care services must offer standards of flexibility and choice in access and quality which match those offered in the private sector. Thus 'the purpose of the 20th century welfare state was to treat citizens as equals, the purpose of 21st century reforms must be to treat them as individuals' (Blair 2002). This derives from Giddens' (2000) concept of the Third Way which has informed both the Clinton and Blair administrations. This involves the welfare state moving from its traditional role of providing security against external risks to a greater emphasis on what Giddens terms positive welfare. This aims to connect autonomy with personal and collective responsibilities, and emphasises the need to provide people with information to inform choices and reduce barriers to access, while accepting that individual choices contribute to inequity in the uptake of health care and health outcomes. Conversely, the shift in thinking in the US was from a market philosophy to a greater emphasis on health care as a public good and universal coverage for services.

Consequences for equity of access

In absolute terms the populations of affluent countries now have access to a considerably increased quantity and range of health care services than in previous decades. Even in market-oriented health systems the provision of basic care is generally available for the poorest groups through publicly funded schemes. However, inequity in terms of relative access to health care tends to increase in this situation of expanding opportunities for treatment unless public policies give priority to this goal in the allocation and distribution of health care resources.

One concern is that even in publicly funded systems, initial access to and uptake of health and medical services may not guarantee equity of access to specialist and high-cost services. Both explicit and more informal rationing increasingly occur in response to cost pressures. As initial access to health care has been achieved, barriers to accessing different levels of care have assumed greater importance. These are exemplified by some of the problems in accessing elective hospital care discussed in Chapter 5. These internal health system barriers to access may encourage an expansion of the private sector thus increasing system and population inequity and the significance of financial barriers (Blendon *et al.* 2002).

The additional opportunities offered through an expansion of consumer choice are more likely to be taken up by more affluent groups and this will also have the effect of compromising equity, and the development of services based on locally expressed needs will introduce inequalities in provision. Equity does not require identical services everywhere. Indeed, differential needs and circumstances may require differential provision. However, inter-locality differences in service provision can mean that people with similar medical conditions differ in the availability of services, as with the so-called 'postcode prescribing' and varying waiting times between different geographic areas in the UK.

The importance assigned to equity of access and the policies implemented to achieve this vary between countries, as Chapters 7 and 8 demonstrate. This reflects wider ideologies and approaches to public policy. Greater emphasis has been given to equity of access to health care in countries with welfare-oriented approaches to public policy compared with those with more market-oriented approaches. There has been a more general adoption of the policy goal of achieving increased efficiency with a more competitive approach to the provision of health care, even in countries that have traditionally relied on publicly funded health care. However, there is 'still no consensus as to how to deal with policies that may cause a conflict between the goals of equity and efficiency' (Sassi *et al.* 2001: 762).

The next chapter in the evolving history of access to health care will be written through the trade-offs made by politicians, managers, clinicians, patients and ultimately by the public, in attempting to reconcile apparently conflicting objectives in providing access to health care. These concern the priorities given to equity or efficiency, solidarity versus individual choice, or universal rights compared with individual responsibility in health care. These decisions will vary for different health conditions and for different population groups. Most choices concerning access will be made on the basis of limited and imperfect information concerning their likely consequences. Research incorporating a range of disciplines, including those represented in this book, is needed to inform these debates. One priority should be to facilitate access to health care for marginalised or excluded groups with limited opportunities for advocacy, few resources, and greater needs for health care.

References

Blair, T. (2002) 'At our best when at our boldest'. Speech by Tony Blair, Prime Minister and Leader of the Labour Party, Labour Party conference, Winter Gardens, Blackpool. Available http://www.labour.org.uk/tbconfspeech/; accessed 3 October 2002.

Blendon, R.J., Schoen, C., DesRoches, C.M., Osborn, R., Scoles, K.L. and Zapert, K. (2002) 'Inequities in health care: a five country survey', *Health Affairs*, 21: 182–91.

Daniels, N. (2000) 'Accountability for reasonableness in private and public health insurance'. In A. Coulter and C. Ham (eds) *The Global Challenge of Health Care Rationing*. Buckingham: Open University Press.

Department of Health (1999) *Patient and Public Involvement in the New NHS*. London: The Stationery Office.

Downing Street Newsroom (2002) *Department of Health Public Service Agreement*. London: 10 Downing Street Newsroom. Available http://www.number-10.gov.uk/output/Page5594.asp; accessed 24 September 2002.

Dozet, A., Lyttkens, C.H. and Nystedt, P. (2002) 'Health care for the elderly: two cases of technology diffusion', *Social Science and Medicine*, 54: 49–64.

Giddens, A. (2000) *The Third Way and its Critics*. Cambridge: Polity Press.

Gilson, L. (1998) 'In defence and pursuit of equity', *Social Science and Medicine*, 47(12): 1891–6.

Guadagnoli, E. and Ward, P. (1998) 'Patient participation in decision-making', *Social Science and Medicine*, 47(3): 329–39.

Ham, C. and Honigsbaum, F. (1998) 'Priority setting and rationing of services'. In R.B. Saltman, J. Figueras and C. Sakellarides (eds) *Critical Challenges for Health Care Reform in Europe*. Buckingham: Open University Press.

Kawachi, I., Marshall, S. and Pearce, N. (1991) Social class inequalities in the decline of coronary heart disease among New Zealand men, 1975–1977 to 1985–1987', *International Journal of Epidemiology*, 20: 393–8.

Klein, R., Day, P. and Redmayne, S. (1995) 'Rationing in the NHS: the dance of the seven veils – in reverse', *British Medical Bulletin*, 51: 769–80.

Klein, R., Day, P. and Redmayne, S. (1996) *Managing Scarcity: Priority Setting and Rationing in the National Health Service*. Buckingham: Open University Press.

Klein, R. and Williams, A. (2000) 'Setting priorities: what is holding us back – inadequate information or inadequate institutions?'. In A. Coulter and C. Ham (eds) *The Global Challenge of Health Care Rationing*. Buckingham: Open University Press.

Lindbladh, E., Lyttkens, C.H., Hanson, B.S., Ostergren, P.O. (1998) 'Equity is out of fashion? An essay on autonomy and health policy in the individualised society', *Social Science and Medicine*, 46: 1017–25.

Lindholm, L., Rosen, M. and Emmelin, M. (1996) 'An epidemiological approach towards measuring the trade off between equity and efficiency in health policy', *Health Policy*, 35: 205–16.

Litva, A., Coast, J., Donovan, J., Eyles, J., Shepherd, M., Tacchi, J., Abelson, J. and Morgan, K. (2002) 'The public is too subjective: public involvement at different levels of health-care decision making', *Social Science and Medicine*, 54: 1825–37.

Maxwell, R.J. (1995) 'Why rationing is on the agenda', *British Medical Bulletin*, 51: 761–8.

Mossialos, E. (1998) 'Regulating expenditure on medicines in European Union countries'. In R.B. Saltman, J. Figueras and C. Sakellarides (eds) *Critical Challenges for Health Care Reform in Europe*. Buckingham: Open University Press.

Mullen, P. (1999) 'Public involvement in health care priority setting: an overview of methods for eliciting values', *Health Expectations*, 2: 222–34.

National Advisory Committee on Core Health and Disability Support services (1998) *The Best of Health 3. Are We Doing the Right Things and Are We Doing Those Things Right?* Wellington: National Health Committee.

National Health Service Management Executive (1992) *Local Voices. The Views of Local People in Purchasing for Health*. London: Department of Health.

Parker, R.A. (1975) 'Social administration and scarcity'. In E. Butterworth and R. Holman (eds) *Social Welfare in Modern Britain*. Glasgow: Collins Fontana.

President's Commission for the Study of Ethical Problems in Medicine and Biomedical and Behavioural Research (1983) *Securing Access to Health Care*. Washington, DC: US Government Printing Office.

Saltman, R.B., Figueras, J., Sakellarides, C. (1998) *Critical Challenges for Health Care Reform in Europe*. Buckingham: Open University Press.

Sassi, F., Le Grande, J. and Archard, L. (2001) 'Equity versus efficiency: a dilemma for the NHS', *British Medical Journal*, 323: 762–3.

Swedish Parliamentary Priorities Commission (1995) *Priorities in health care*, Stockholm, Sweden: Ministry of Health & Social Affairs.

Thatcher, M. (1987) 'Aids, education and the year 2000', *Woman's Own*, 3 October 1987: 8–10. Quoted at http://www.cooperativeindividualism.org/thatcher_society_and_responsibility.html; accessed 3 October 2002.

van de Ven, W.P.M. (1995) 'Choices in health care: a contribution from the Netherlands', *British Medical Bulletin*, 51:781–90.

Wanless, D. (2002) *Securing Our Future Health: Taking a Long Term View. Final Report.* London: Her Majesty's Treasury.

Working Group on Health Care Prioritisation (1995) *From Values to Choice.* Helsinki: National Research and Development Centre for Welfare and Health.

Index